Conversation Repair

Conversation Repair

Case Studies in Doctor-Patient Communication

Frederic W. Platt, M.D.

Foreword by
J. Gregory Carroll, Ph.D.

Little, Brown and Company
Boston   New York   Toronto   London

Library of Congress Cataloging-in-Publication Data

Platt, Frederic W.
    Conversation repair / Frederic W. Platt ; foreword by Gregory Carroll
      p.   cm.
    Sequel to: Conversation failure / Frederic W. Platt. ©1994.
    Includes bibliographical references and index.
    ISBN 0-316-71082-2
    1. Physician and patient—Case studies.   2. Medical history taking—Case studies.   I. Platt, Frederic W. Conversation failure. II. Title.
    [DNLM: 1. Communication—case studies.   2. Physician-Patient Relations—case studies.   3. Interviews—case studies.   W 62 P7185c 1995]
    R727.3.P496   1995
    610.69'6—dc20
    DNLM/DLC   95-835
    for Library of Congress   CIP

Printed in the United States of America

CCP

Editorial: Tammerly Booth

Copyeditor: Debra Corman

Production Services and Typesetting: Pageworks

To the physicians who care for patients and who must struggle daily with difficult conversations;

To my parents, Betty and Ben Platt, who encouraged me to enter this work;

and

To the memory of my father-in-law, Harold McCormick, a fine man whom I never had to please and always did.

Contents

4 So What Else Is New? 101

5 The Database 117

6 The Doctor Did It 139

7 Patience, Humility, and Compassion 169

Epilogue 185

References 187

Index 193

Foreword

From my perspective, *Conversation Repair* has a deceptively clear theme, one that probably offends the conventional beliefs of many physicians in practice today. The theme I see is that in extreme cases, doctors seem to communicate as their own worst enemies. Their assumptions, experience, and professional contexts sometimes mislead them into frustrations, dead ends, and conflicts. To make matters worse, the physician often attributes this situation to a "difficult patient."

By reviewing these difficult interactions and reframing them as both curiosities and challenges, Dr. Fred Platt attacks the longstanding assumption that certain doctors are natural communicators while others are not. He demonstrates how some specific communication skills, such as discovering patients' meaning and paraphrasing their beliefs, can dramatically reduce or prevent many of these frustrations and conflicts. He also elicits the reader's empathy for the physician's dilemma in such cases. What is a doctor to do?

An important factor in the book's effectiveness, as well as the reader's enjoyment, is that *Conversation Repair* was written as a series of case discussions rather than as a conventional text on doctor-patient communication. Skills, principles, and techniques are introduced and illustrated in the context of real life cases drawn from medical practice. The cases are not intended to represent a typical day's schedule. Rather, they focus attention on types of communication disasters that sometimes occur.

Each section of the book concentrates on a specific set of skills. An effective way to test and apply these skills is to reflect on each case and think about each question that the author raises. How would you be inclined to respond? What would you do? What would you say? How would you say it? Above all, try to remain flexible as a reader and imagine different paths that might have different results. How do your responses compare with those quoted in the text or with those suggested by the author? What factors in your experience or your assumptions might account for these differences?

Dr. Fred Platt joined the workshop faculty of the Miles Institute for Health Care Communication* in 1990. As a teacher, writer, and clinician he has contributed significantly to our understanding and our curriculum on physician-patient communication, especially the "Difficult" Physician-Patient Relationships workshop. On behalf of the Institute, I would like to acknowledge our profound respect, appreciation, and affection for Fred as a colleague and friend.

Conversation Repair is great testimony to Fred's insight and to his professional commitment to the field of health care communication. This book is also a wonderful reflection of the collaboration that takes place within the Institute's faculty. I am enormously grateful to Fred for all of the above.

J. Gregory Carroll, Ph.D.

*As of April 1995, the Miles Institute for Health Care Communication will change its name to the Bayer Institute for Health Care Communication.

Preface

Conversation Repair contains 53 doctor-patient dialogues. Each is problematic, usually unsatisfactory to doctor and patient alike. Following each dialogue I have posed questions that seem germane to the difficulty. I suggest that the reader stop and consider what he or she thinks is going on and what would be the best tactic to get things back on an even keel. Only then would I recommend reading on.

In each case I have attempted to describe a route out of that particular difficulty. There are certainly other, perhaps better, routes to success that I could not see at the time. In some cases there may not be a best route, and we seldom know at the time what will work best. But my thesis is this: *Disasters and difficulties occur often in doctor-patient conversations. It is our job to recognize them, sort them out, and attempt to repair them. Conversation repair is as essential as the diagnosis and therapy of organic disease if one is to be a real doctor.*

Conversation Repair is a sequel to a previous book, *Conversation Failure: Case Studies in Doctor-Patient Communication.* Since our communication disasters don't come to us in any particular order, I intentionally scrambled the cases in that first book. In *Conversation Repair*, I have made an effort to group the cases in seven categories: Discover Meaning, Effective Empathy, Acknowledgment, So What Else Is New?, The Database, The Doctor Did It, and Patience, Humility, and Compassion. Each section of this book begins with a discussion of the sort of problem to be encountered in that section and the generic solution I recommend for that problem. But, because all of the cases are real and have the confusing mixture of reality, they resist precise categorization. A case included under the category Discover Meaning might just as easily have been placed in the category Effective Empathy. In fact, since each category really defines a therapeutic approach to treating conversation failure, it should be no surprise that different therapies will often help the same disordered interview.

To the reader, I suggest an open attitude. Some of the techniques that I advise may seem foreign or unlikely. As you try them, you may find that your application feels wooden or mechanical. Don't worry. After practice, the techniques will seem easy and useful. Pretty soon your colleagues will watch you with awe and will describe you as "born to communicate." Only you need know the truth.

The cases cited come from several sources, including my own practice. In those situations, I tried to re-create the dialogue as soon after hearing it as I could. I realize that I might be guilty of some unconscious editing, but I have not tried to hide my own error or failures. Instead, I have tried to expose them to scrutiny.

Some of the dialogues were recorded while observing house staff at Presbyterian/Saint Luke's Medical Center in Denver, where I have been teaching students and house staff for 20 years. Other dialogues were reported to me by physicians at Miles workshops or over a lunch table. A few came from my colleague, Dr. A. Lee Anneberg. In most of the cases told to me by another physician, the story was prefaced by "You won't believe what happened to me yesterday." One might wonder about the accuracy of reporting in this group. Can physicians be trusted to recount a dialogue this way? Probably not entirely. Doctors don't remember exactly what the patient said, and they remember even less of what they themselves said. But the interactions these doctors report are often poignant. In a few cases the doctor could not forget the interaction for years. For example, the first case in this book took place a year before the doctor recounted it to us. He was unsure of some of the actual dialogue but very sure of the overall process and its terrible outcome.

There is a vast literature dealing with doctor-patient communication. I have made no attempt to cite it systematically. However, I have not been able to resist including a handful of favorite references when they seemed especially pertinent.

I have great respect for the physicians who engage in the work of clinical care of patients. It takes courage and stamina to do this work. I dedicate this book to all such physicians.

F.P.

Acknowledgments

This book is a sequel to *Conversation Failure: Case Studies in Doctor-Patient Communication,* published in 1992 by Life Sciences Press, to whom I owe a debt for their encouragement.

I have been stumbling over, studying, and sorting out disordered interviews for 20 years, but I believe that my understanding of these problems has been aided considerably in the last five years by the work being done by the Miles Institute for Health Care Communication. The staff of that institute has taught me a great deal. The categorization of cases in this book reflects the therapeutic techniques that they teach in the Miles workshops on doctor-patient communication and the difficult physician-patient relationship. I want to acknowledge a great debt to the Miles Institute for Health Care Communication and especially to Greg Carroll and Vaughn Keller of the institute for their continual support, encouragement, and helpful coaching.

Many of these cases came from my own practice and that of my colleague, Dr. A. Lee Anneberg. I owe a great deal to Lee for his helpful discussions of my own failed communication and for his courageous willingness to contribute some of his own very difficult cases. Lee is a superb clinician. When he struggles with an interaction, we can be sure of its difficulty; I feel fortunate to be able to use them as examples.

Several cases were donated by other physicians. I want to thank Drs. Elisabet Atkin-Thor, David Beck, Bradd Christensen, Ted Clarke, Dennis Conrad, Bryce Fairbanks, Geoffrey Gordon, Jerry Hammon, Tim Hopf, Gamil Kostandy, Robert Parsons, Robert Shubinsky, Jonathan Singer, Bruce Williams, and Ms. Jane Monaghan for their stories.

Several of these interactions have already been published. I thank *Vital Facts* for permission to reprint The Kidney Stone and Burning in My Stomach. I thank *Patient Care* magazine for permission to reprint Kathleen, Are you Grieving; What's My Hemoglobin; Hyperbole, Indeed; Nosy Doctor; The Treacherous K-Y Jelly Disaster; Will He Get Better?; It All Began in 1949; It's Hard Not to Smoke; I'm Sick, Doctor; Choking to Death; Boulder Knee; I'm Not Talking; Tomorrow; I Hope I Answered Your Questions All Right; and Not Fit for a Human Being. Much of the discussion in the introduction to Effective Empathy first appeared in the *Journal of General Internal Medicine* [17], and much of the discussion in The Doctor Did It first appeared in *The Annals of Internal Medicine* [10].

Lisa Logan and Greg Carroll have read the manuscript and helped to clarify my own confusion and that of my writing. I appreciate their help and encouragement.

Most of all, I want to thank Connie Platt. She has stood by me for 37 years, has offered support and helpful ideas when I felt burdened by the difficulties my patients presented, and has been enormously helpful in editing this very manuscript. I want to explain the nature of her editorial help. She has not only asked me if "this is the way you want to say it," but often if "this is what you would really prefer to say or do with your patients." Thus, her editing included coaching in the art of doctoring as well as that of writing. Since this book is partly a self-exploration, Connie's editorial guidance has often been helpful at self-discovery and self-understanding. I cannot thank her enough.

1

Discover Meaning

Why does he keep telling me about his long-dead Uncle Louis?

Dr. X

When in doubt, be curious.

Vaughn Keller

We must take our students where we find them and lead them where they are willing to go.

Barbara Korsch, M.D.

Our job isn't to know, but to find out.

Mack Lipkin, Jr., M.D.

Consider this brief dialogue:

Dr. X: How long have you had the chest pain?
Mr. Y: Since I moved to Denver.
X: And how long ago was that?
Y: About three years.

We all experience similar conversations every day. The doctor is wondering what he has to do to get his patient to answer simple questions. The patient may be frustrated because his doctor seems to have so little interest in what the patient

1

sees as most important, the connection between his pain and his move to Denver. The doctor silently complains to himself, "Another person who insists on telling stories instead of answering questions." The patient, trying to help his doctor, moves into the doctor's framework and clarifies the time interval.

Elliot Mishler [1] defines two languages, that of doctors and that of patients. He says that doctors speak in a language of medicine, stressing facts, measurable intervals and sizes, sequences and events. Our patients speak primarily in the language of the life world, stressing relationships and causes. Most of all our patients want to understand *why* they are suffering as they are, and when they have a theory about this *why*, they want to share it with us. Thus when we ask our patient for a time interval, expecting an answer in hours or days, months or years, we shouldn't be surprised that the patient answers an entirely different question, one that seems more paramount to him: "Why are you having this symptom? What do you surmise might be connected to it causally?" To the patient in the previous dialogue, the why has to do with the move to Denver. If you asked him how the two were connected, he might admit that he didn't know but that he came to you to find out. Nonetheless, he has noted the connection between the move and the pain and doesn't want you to miss it.

Mishler says that we have to deal with both languages to be humane doctors. He thinks we should at least let our patient know that we have heard him before insisting that he enter our world, speak our language, and answer our question. We might at least acknowledge his statement in our revised question, "I see. You've had this pain since you moved to Denver. And how long ago was that?"

Arthur Kleinman [2] says that we do pretty well in defining diseases but that we often misunderstand illness. He says that we want to "arrange for therapeutic manipulation of the disease problems in place of a meaningful moral response to illness problems." He recommends that we try to understand the meaning of the illness to the patient and that to do so we should ask what the illness has done to his life, to his hopes, his work, and his family. What is his understanding of the disease and how does he view his caregivers? What does he fear next from the disease? What is left of the person he once was?

The doctor-patient relationship, fundamentally like any other human relationship, has to be built on understanding if it is to succeed. I am sure that we fail most often in understanding. Surely we lack at times in explaining our ideas and our plans. Surely our patients need more explanation and more education from us. But much more often it is we who lack an adequate understanding. If we knew where our patients were "coming from," we'd be better at helping them to move to where they want to go. I believe that Barbara Korsch is right about our students, and the same stipulation would hold for our patients. If we are to lead them anywhere, first we have to find out where they are. That may take a lot of finding out.

So what do we need to understand? No list will suffice for all patients, and there will always be more to know than we can possibly learn in our limited time with the patient, but here are some considerations:

1. What sort of person is this: one who says little and bears his suffering silently or one who asks for help easily?

2. What makes up this person's world—people, work, major interests and worries? What has made up his world in the past? What are his joys and his sorrows?

3. What important past influences color the patient's view of the present?

4. What is this illness doing to the patient's life? To his work, relationships, hopes for the future, self-definition?

5. What does the patient think caused this illness? What sort of guilt and responsibility does she think she bears?

6. What are the symptoms of the illness? What are their parameters (where, when, how bad, what makes it better or worse, associated symptoms, and so on)?

7. What have other people told the patient about his illness? What other diagnostic, etiologic, and therapeutic considerations does he have?

8. What does the patient hope you will do for her? What does she expect? What are her other concerns?

Are we ever likely to know all this? Perhaps not quickly. But we can bet that if we suffer a disruption in our relationship, it will be the result of misunderstanding how the patient perceives his or her situation. Sometimes we can best learn what we need to know by asking a generic sort of question during the interview: "Is there something else I need to know to understand you and your illness?"

More often the puzzling area is clearly demarcated, and we can be more precise: "I can see that you really don't want to go to the hospital. But I haven't yet understood your concerns or fears. Can you help me understand better?"

I agree with Mack Lipkin. Our job isn't to know, but to find out. And there's a lot more to find out than we usually include in our disease-oriented database.

The concept that encountering the patient and his or her illness is a process of discovering meaning can serve as a guideline for all our interviews. For some of us, Discovering Meaning can be a mantra to focus our approach. Every encounter described in this book illustrates the process or the results of neglecting to discover meaning.

John Berger [3] describes understanding in terms of brotherhood:

> He should recognize his patient with the certainty of an ideal brother. The function of fraternity is recognition. . . . This individual and closely intimate recognition is required on both a physical and psychological level. On the former it constitutes the art of diagnosis. . . . On the psychological level recognition means support.

Case 1

I NEED AN ANTIBIOTIC

Dr. X works at a walk-in clinic that is well equipped for emergency and urgent care but not for continuing care. A 59-year-old man arrives requesting an antibiotic.

X: Hello, Mr. Grave. I'm Dr. X. What can I do for you?

G: I just need an antibiotic. I've got a leg infection. Shouldn't be much.

X: OK. Who is your usual doctor?

G: I don't go to doctors. I haven't had a doctor for 20 years. I don't believe in 'em.

X: Uh huh. And besides your leg, are you having any other trouble?

G: Nah. Maybe a little trouble with my wind. I don't breathe as well as I used to. It's probably just the cigarettes.

X: I see. And how many cigarettes is that?

G: Not so much. I smoke about two packs a day, but mostly they just burn out in the ashtray.

X: OK. Well, since I've never seen you before, how about if you strip down to your shorts and I'll do an examination?

G: It's just my leg.

X: Well, the leg is attached to the rest of you, so let me look a little more carefully.

The examination was a surprise to Dr. X. His patient had basilar rales on both sides of his chest, poor breath sounds throughout, elevated venous pressure, a big liver, and four-plus leg edema. The legs were so edematous that fluid was weeping through the skin. Dr. X did some laboratory studies. Mr. G was mildly hypoxic with an oxygen saturation of 88%, had congested lungs on the chest x-ray, and was erythrocytotic. Dr. X thought that his patient had cigarette-induced chronic obstructive lung disease with secondary heart failure and hypoxia. He thought that hospitalization was the answer.

X: Well, Mr. G, I think that your trouble is more than an infected leg. In fact, I think the swelling in your legs is part of a condition of fluid retention throughout your body. We call it heart failure, and I think we have to get you into the hospital to help you out.

G: No.

X: What?

G: No. I ain't going.

X: To the hospital?

G: Yeah. I came for an antibiotic. That's all.

X: Even if I think that's not the trouble or the solution?

G: Yeah.

X: Well, then. Hmm. What . . ., who. . . . Did you come here with anyone else?

G: Yeah, my wife.

X: Can I talk with her?

G: OK.

The doctor asked a nurse to bring the patient's wife into the examination room. Soon the conversation included three participants.

X: Mrs. G, we're stuck here. Your husband needs to go to the hospital and doesn't want to.

Mrs. G: I was afraid of that.

G: I ain't going.

Mrs. G: He's bullheaded. I can't ever make him do anything he doesn't want to do.

X: It's the only way we can help.

G: Then I'll just go home.

X: It's really too complicated to try to treat your heart failure as an outpatient. We're not set up for good follow-up care here.

G: That's fine, Doc. If you can't give me an antibiotic, that's OK.

X: I really think you have to come into the hospital, Mr. G. You're not well, and we need to take care of this. You aren't going to get well at home without a lot of help.

G: Doc, you decide what you do, and I decide what I do. I'm going home.

This patient and his wife left the emergent-care unit and went home. The doctor felt frustrated by his inability to persuade his patient to do otherwise. However, as usual in that clinic, he planned to call the patient in 48 hours for a follow-up.

• What would you say is at the heart of this impasse?

- What do you do when you are at loggerheads with your patient?
- What would you do now?

Discussion

At the heart of this standoff is a difference of opinion. The doctor and his patient disagree on diagnosis and on therapy. They are at an impasse. Mr. G has diagnosed his problem as an infected leg, and he is confident he knows how to fix it. He believes he is a better diagnostician than the guy with the credentials, which at this point seems beyond Dr. X's ability to imagine.

And there is a struggle for control. Who is really in charge of Mr. G's fate? Mr. G has some strong opinions on that score. Dr. X is not going to get anywhere with Mr. G until he understands who's the boss.

This patient may also have some strong feelings about hospitalization that are so far unclarified. Is he afraid? What has happened to him in the past in hospitals? What has happened to other people he knows? The doctor could try to discover the reasons for his reluctance. Greg Carroll recommends asking the patient more specifically about the meaning of the word *hospital* from his own experience. Discovering the patient's view of the hospital may uncover the reasons for his reluctance. If he tried this approach the doctor might have heard something like this:

X: Gosh! It sounds like going to the hospital is the last thing you want to do.
G: Yeah.
X: What's that about? Something bad happened to you before in a hospital?
G: No, not to me. I don't go near 'em.
X: But?
G: But what?

[Silence.]

G: Well, my brother died in one. They cut him up and that was it.

Mrs. G: That's not true, he had bad heart trouble first. It wasn't their fault.

X: Still, that's the way hospitals look to you.

G: Yeah.

Once the patient's picture of his situation was clearer, Dr. X may have been able to negotiate:

X: Well, we're still stuck. I'm pretty sure that we can do best for you in the hospital. Are you sure you won't go in?

G: Yeah, Doc. I'm sure. If I'm going to die, I'd rather do it at home.

X: Well, I don't think hospitals are just for dying. Is that how it looks to you?

G: That's it, Doc. No hospitals.

X: OK. What if we tried some medicine first at home? Then you could come back here, say, in a day or two, and we could see if we'd made any change. We still might have to say then that the hospital was the place. How will you feel if that's where we end up?

G: What kind of medicine?

X: I think we would best start with a heart-strengthening medicine, digoxin, and a diuretic to help you shed excess water. Both are pills you could take.

G: Well, I could try the medicine first. Maybe if it didn't help, we could talk. Will you be here in two days?

Too far-fetched? Maybe. We won't know because no negotiated settlement was reached.

When the doctor phoned two days later, he learned, to his horror, that the patient had a "big argument" with his wife the day after his medical visit, went out to his backyard with a pistol, shot himself, and was now dead.

This event occurred one year ago, and the doctor is still distressed by it, still asking himself what else he might have done, and still feeling guilty about the result. Is there more to say?

One colleague suggested to me that when the patient refuses to do what we recommend, it makes sense to ask him what he plans to do instead. Maybe, just maybe, such a question would have revealed the suicidal considerations. If it had, perhaps Dr. X could have made some further efforts to intervene.

When the doctor recounted this story, I suggested that he might allay some of his feelings of guilt by extending care to Mrs. G, the patient's wife. She too probably still has a lot of sadness, anger, and guilt about her husband's death. It wouldn't be too late, even now, to call her and say that he was "thinking about Mr. G and his last illness and suicide a year ago." He could tell her that he was thinking of how hard it must be for her, ask how she has handled it and how her last year has been. Such a call could be a real gift to her, and since giving a gift always lightens our burdens, it might lighten his.

Case 2

I'M REALLY UPSET

The patient, a 55-year-old woman, had consulted Dr. X because of increasing cough and dyspnea. She had a two-year history of asthma and said that she was using inhaled bronchodilators and steroids. Dr. X carefully reviewed her history and examined her. The examination was entirely normal, including her chest.

Four months later she returned, telling again of increasing cough. She admitted not using the inhaled medications at all. After his examination, Dr. X spent 20 minutes carefully instructing her on proper use of the medications, writing out all his instructions.

One week later she called, saying she was better, but had not filled her prescriptions. The very next day she appeared again at the office, now admitting to six months of cough, even occasional hemoptysis, but reported that she still had not taken her medicines. Dr. X was annoyed.

Dr. X: I am really upset! I went to the trouble to write down all my instructions, and you haven't followed any of them!

Ms. P: [Standing and crying] I want to leave. I want to go.

X: Well, wait a minute. I'm sorry to upset you. But I do want you to know that you are not following my advice. You asked for my advice and didn't follow it.

P: [Sniffling] OK, I will try. What do you want me to do?

Dr. X arranged for a CT scan of the sinuses and a chest x-ray, called her the next day with the results (diffuse mucosal sinus thickening), and recommended a nasal steroid. She was to return in one week. One day before that visit she called to cancel and said that she didn't want to reschedule.

Asked about the interchange, Dr. X said, "Sometimes I thought she wasn't really listening to me. She sat and stared at her lap and remained silent. She never looked at me."

When asked how he came to get angry with her, Dr. X said, "I had spent a lot of extra time writing it all out, and she acted as if my work wasn't worth anything."

- What WAS Ms. P listening to?
- What triggers your anger? Do you get angry when your advice is disregarded by your patient? What do you do then?

Discussion

Dr. X doesn't get angry easily, and when he does, he seldom shows it openly. About the most he might admit to is "being upset." But we can bet that he was angry this time and that his patient felt the anger. Although the relationship seemed to return to an even keel, the patient's failure to come back probably implies the existence of an unresolved issue. And of course the initial puzzle still remains: Why was this patient coming to the doctor for advice and then not following it?

I think the doctor's observation that his patient seemed not to be listening to him could lead us to an approach that might work.

X: You know, Ms. P, as I talk I notice that you seem to be thinking of something else. Is there a concern or worry you have that I don't even know about?

Until we find out what she IS listening to, we won't know why she isn't able to hear us.

What about the doctor's anger? Many of us find it hard to bear when patients disregard our advice. We interpret this as disrespect and may take it personally. This is doctor-centered thinking that may stem from our own insecurities about self-worth. We may feel victimized at such a point and, becoming angry, think to ourselves: "This patient isn't thinking of me at all. She doesn't consider my feelings. She just cares about herself, and she is wasting my valuable time. Why doesn't she just find a friend to talk to if she doesn't plan to follow my advice?"

A better approach is to remember that the patient's actions are not directed at us and they tell us something about her, but what? We can find out by taking care to identify the problem as our faulty understanding, not her noncompliance.

X: Ms. P, I notice that you haven't taken the medicines I recommended and are feeling worse. Can you help me understand what's going on?

A straightforward and pure description of our ignorance is essential. We must take great care not to mix in our theories about the patient's feelings and ideas until we really know what they are.

Adherence cannot be assumed. We have to enlist the patient, and when she fails in so spectacular a way, we should take it as a message: There is something here that we don't yet understand. Maybe she's more afraid of the treatment than of the disease. Maybe she is in full-fledged denial that she is really sick. Maybe she is frightened by another diagnosis she is considering—lung cancer or tuberculosis, AIDS or whatever. The big truth is that we DO NOT YET KNOW what is going through this patient's mind, and so we can't help her. We must first solve the communication problem before we can do more for her asthma.

Case 3

NOT LOOKING

Mrs. J is 84 years old and has been hospitalized for congestive heart failure. She suddenly developed atrial fibrillation with a rapid ventricular rate and heart failure. An electrocardiogram disclosed a new inferior myocardial infarction. Treated with digitalis, diuretics, and angiotensin-converting enzyme inhibitors, she seemed to be doing well in the hospital, but today, seven days after admission, she seems different.

Dr. X: Well, how are you doing today, Selma?

Ms. R (a nurse, trying to help the patient with her lunch): She seems worse somehow. She won't eat, and she won't open her eyes.

X: I see that. What's the trouble, Selma? That looks like a tasty lunch.

S: I'm not hungry.

X: I see. And why are you keeping your eyes closed?

[Silence.]

X: Selma, do you know who I am?

S: Of course. You're my doctor. You're Dr. X.

X: Yes. And why are your eyes closed? Can you open them?

[She opens her eyes briefly, glances at the doctor, then closes them.]

X: What's going on?

[Prolonged silence.]

S: Father R was in and gave me last rites.

X: Yes?

[Silence.]

X: Selma, do you think you are going to die?

[Pause.]

S: Yes.
X: I see.

[Pause.]

X: But I still don't understand the closed eyes.

[Silence.]

S: I don't want to look.
X: Not look?
S: I don't want to see it happen.
X: You don't want to see yourself die?
S: That's right.
X: I see. So you had last rites, and now you think you have to die and you're keeping your eyes closed so you won't see it happen.
S: That's right [opening her eyes and staring at the doctor].
X: Well, actually I don't think you are just about to die. I hope that isn't disappointing to you.
S: No it isn't [chuckling a little]. What's for lunch?

- What accounts for this conversational miracle?
- Did you have any other theories about her closed eyes?

Discussion

Amazing? I think so. Sometimes it all falls out very logically if we can just take our time and think about what we are seeing and hearing. We must remember that the patient always has a reason for beliefs and behavior. Getting her to share it is our challenge.

Making use of silence helps. If we observe acutely, then ask the right question, we still have to wait for an answer. Pausing long enough to allow the patient to find that answer is hard. Nature and doctors abhor a vacuum; we rush to fill silences. It works better if we can trust the silence to do its work.

Finally, I can't really explain some of these conversational miracles. Much of what works best is an unconscious empathy, a true feeling-with. When that happens I am content to enjoy the interaction and be grateful for the miracle.

Case 4

NOW WE CAN DO WHAT I WANT

The patient was a meek 60-year-old woman who came to see her husband's orthopedist. Her husband acted as spokesman and explained that she was suffering with low back pain. She was able to describe her symptoms but was quite subdued. The orthopedist examined her and thought she had the usual sort of lumbar backache.

Dr. D: Well, you seem to have a musculoskeletal backache, all right. I don't think the pain is referred from anything inside, and I see no evidence that the trouble is interfering with normal neurological function. I think that we can help you. I'm going to give you some medicine, what we call a nonsteroidal anti-inflammatory drug, and I want you to get some physical therapy.

Mrs. Meek: OK, Doctor.

D: I will have my assistant arrange for you to go to the physical therapy department. Then I'd like to see you again in two weeks.

M: OK, Doctor.

Two weeks later the couple returned. Now the tables seemed turned. The husband was meek and subdued and his wife triumphant.

Mrs. M: Doctor, I did what you said. I took the pills, and I went to the therapist. And I'm not one whit better. I'm exactly the same!

The physician examined her, found no new abnormalities, and said so.

D: I'm sorry you're still hurting, Mrs. M. I don't find any new abnormalities on my examination though.

M: Well I've tried what you two wanted. Now I can do what I wanted. I'm going to my chiropractor. He'll put my back right. Thank you for your efforts, Doctor. I know what I need, and I'm going to get it.

With that, she marched out of the office, followed, at a respectful distance, by her husband.

- Was there anything at the first visit that might have alerted Dr. D?
- Was anything left undone at the first visit that might have helped?

Discussion

Dr. D says that he thinks it would have helped if he had said less and listened more. He thinks he might have asked Mrs. M what she thought was wrong and what she thought might be most helpful. Perhaps if he had done so at the first visit, she would have told him that she thought her back was "out of alignment" and that a chiropractor would help more than his suggested approach. If so, Dr. D says, he would have suggested that she do just that, consult a chiropractor and perhaps try a few treatments, just not sign up for a complete course of 20 or 30 visits.

I think Dr. D has the right idea about asking his patient for her own diagnosis and her own idea of correct therapy. Then I think he could offer her a reasonable choice.

D: I see. You think this is a bad alignment problem and that a chiropractor might be able to manipulate it and fix it.

M: Yes.

D: Well, I can understand your choosing that strategy. Perhaps you could try the chiropractor for a couple of visits, then, if everything isn't fine, come back here. Or, you might first try some medication that I could prescribe, use a heating pad, and physical therapy. It's your choice.

M: He [pointing to her husband] doesn't think my chiropractor can help.

D: Well, I think we often do better, but some people get relief from chiropractic manipulations. And of course lots of people get better whatever we do.

M: I'm glad to hear you say that, Doctor. OK. What if I just try your ideas first? When did you want me back?

With such an interchange, I suspect that Dr. D's therapy would stand a better chance at success, and the face-off between Mrs. M and her husband about therapeutic alternatives would not have to continue.

Discovering meaning often leads us far from what we usually consider to be orthopedics. But sometimes the missing understanding is simple—just what did the patient think was wrong and what did she think we should do about it?

Case 5

KATHLEEN, ARE YOU GRIEVING

Kathleen first came to see me two years ago at the age of 38. At that time she felt well except for fatigue and right-sided numbness that came and went over a 16-month period. The fatigue usually increased as the day progressed. Neither symptom interfered with her work or vigorous athletics. She had consulted several neurologists and had been studied with cerebral CT and MRI. The neurological examinations had been normal, but the MR scan had shown some high-intensity foci in white matter of both hemispheres. She understood that the diagnosis was unclear but that her symptoms might indicate the presence of a demyelinating disease, perhaps multiple sclerosis. Fortunately, the symptoms gradually faded, and within half a year she was back to her usual strength and energy, no longer bothered by hemihypesthesia.

A year ago Kathleen felt fine when she appeared for her annual physical examination, but one week ago she again developed right-sided numbness. A repeat physical examination was normal except for some vague decrease in sensation in her right arm and leg. The repeat MR scan was unchanged from two years ago.

She left the office in her usual cheerful mood, promising to call back after she returned from a weekend jaunt to Las Vegas, but yesterday she called in tears. The trip had been "terrible." She was "having a terrible time; losing it; crying all the time." Her mouth was cottony, and there was a lump stuck in her throat.

When she appeared at the office, she said that she was frightened, that "the uncertainty was weighing" on her. She said that her husband was very concerned and hoped for a clearer answer. Then she explained that she was usually "not like this."

Kathleen: I'm not like this. [Weeping] I don't cry. I don't even know why I'm crying. I'm usually the calm one. In my family I'm the one who holds everything together.

Dr. P: You're not one to smear your mascara?

K: Exactly! I like to be the one to take care of the others. I'm really quite cheerful. I don't lose control like this.

P: It sounds as if you're sad, even grieving.

K: Yes. But why? What would I be grieving about? Nothing different has really happened. And it's not work or home. Things are going fine at work, except I have a friend who reads a lot—she thinks maybe I have a yeast problem or EB virus trouble. And home is fine. My husband is very concerned.

P: So you are caught in an uncertain situation, knowing that it might all get better again or that it could possibly deteriorate.

K: Yes.

P: And your work friend has all sorts of diagnoses to try out on you.

K: Yes [laughing].

P: And your husband wants more certainty, too.

K: Yes.

P: And worst of all, you seem to be full of sadness and you don't know why.

K: That's it. I'm just not like this usually. I'm sorry that I'm breaking down here. Please pardon my tears. [Crying] I'm not like this.

• What do you think? Why is Kathleen crying?

Discussion

Gerard Manley Hopkins explained grief in his short poem, "Spring and Fall" [4]:

SPRING AND FALL: TO A YOUNG CHILD

Margaret, are you grieving
Over Goldengrove unleaving?
Leaves, like the things of man, you
With your fresh thoughts care for, can you?
Ah! as the heart grows older
It will come to such sights colder
By and by, nor spare a sigh
Though worlds of wanwood leafmeal lie;
And yet you WILL weep and know why.
Now no matter, child, the name:
Sorrow's springs are the same.
Nor mouth had, no nor mind, expressed
What heart heard of, ghost guessed:
It is the blight man was born for,
It is Margaret you mourn for.

Does that help? Or does it just confuse matters more? The real cause of grief, Hopkins believes, is our sense of loss when we realize the inevitability of our own death. We weep for ourselves.

Under the threat of a diagnosis of multiple sclerosis, Kathleen may be grieving her own potential loss of hopes and possibilities. I think this illness has momentarily gone past her defenses, to be cheerful, contained, and to care for others. These powerful and admirable traits have been overwhelmed, and for a moment she is face-to-face with her own mortality. It is Kathleen for whom she mourns.

Grieving is difficult for Kathleen, who is usually optimistic; her grief may be equally difficult for her physician, who has come to like and admire her noncomplaining style. We tend to like people who are competent, self-contained, and cheerful. When they lose their composure, we too may feel the loss. But it is not their job to "take care" of us. We have to be able to bear their pain and their sadness in order to support them as they experience those feelings.

What might the physician say after understanding his patient's grief? I like the short responses: "Oh! I understand!" or "I see. Yes, now I understand better."

Case 6

MY SON IS IN A SITUATION

The doctor was called to the phone to talk to Mrs. B.

Dr. X: Hello, this is Dr. Xylom.

B: Hello, Doctor. Thank you for taking my call. I need to talk with you. I think I told you last time that I was under a lot of stress. It's about my son. He's in a situation.

X: Hmm. I don't remember your mentioning that. Tell me more about it.

B: Well, he was with some friends in a car, and someone shot at them.

X: Oh my goodness. Is he all right?

B: Yes, well someone else in the car handed him a gun, and by accident he shot it out the window and someone else was hit. The other person was hurt, he was badly, he was . . . that is, he is dead.

X: Your son shot and killed someone?

B: Yes. And he's in that place, and they've had their psychiatrists see him.

X: In jail?

B: Yes. And they think he's bipolar, and they want a private psychiatrist to see him.

X: How terrible for you! This must be just awful for you. He's your only son?

B: Yes. My son is in a situation. And I need the name of a psychiatrist.

X: Someone outside of the police department to evaluate him?

B: Yes. This all happened in April.

X: Two months ago? That was before you were in for your physical examination. Did you tell me about all this then?

B: No, I just mentioned that I was a little stressed out about my children.

X: More than your son?

B: No, just him. He's in a situation.

- What do you think of this euphemism?
- Why didn't Mrs. B tell the doctor earlier about her son?

Discussion

The Major General in Gilbert and Sullivan's *Pirates of Penzance* explains that he "had to tell a story" (a falsehood), but that it wasn't as bad as a "regular story" because he had a good excuse [5]. We color our stories to make them seem better to us and our listeners. Snyder et al. [6] explain that the function of excuses is to shade reality to a tone that we can stand. If we have a hard time being seen or seeing ourselves as we are, we use excuses to put ourselves in a better light. We may spend much of our time attempting to reedit the past, rather than addressing the present or the future.

Mrs. B is not ready yet to talk about the enormity of her son's action. Calling it "a situation" minimizes the problem to a size she can deal with. She may also feel some shame at being the mother of a murderer, and the euphemism deflects that.

Why didn't Mrs. B mention her son's arrest when she saw the doctor two months ago? She tried to, but he didn't understand. When she reported that she was "a little stressed out" about her children, a request for details might have elicited the whole story. At some level, perhaps the doctor knew there was a "story" behind her remark and didn't want to ask about it.

Why? Maybe the usual pressure of time. It seems to us that we can get by on partial understanding and that more understanding demands more time than we have allocated to that patient's visit.

Our patients come to us with all kinds of pain, and although we may not have realized it when we went to medical school, receiving the pain is what we signed up for. We have to ask so we can respond to the whole of the patient's life. The doctor's response to the phone call is a model of kindness. He clarifies the situation, empathizes with the patient, and will be able to help her with a referral and support.

2

Effective Empathy

I can't cope with patients who are irrational. If they're teary or angry, they can just come back another time.

Dr. X

The only thing we learned about King Alfred was about him burning the cakes."
"That's something though, isn't it? It's a fact —
perhaps *it's a fact. But they don't go in for facts in History these days. They go in for empathy, Lewis. Whatever that is."*
"What's the drill then, sir?"

Colin Dexter [7]

In 1989, Vaughn Keller, now associate director of the Miles Institute for Health Care Communication in West Haven, Connecticut, developed a half-day communication workshop for practicing physicians [8]. Since 1990 the workshop has been conducted over 500 times for more than 8,000 doctors. This Physician-Patient Communication Workshop begins with a "frustration exercise." The doctors are asked to name and describe their most frustrating patient or doctor-patient encounter [9]. Later they work in groups to recreate the dialogues from these frustrating experiences.

We have found a remarkable consistency in the kinds of encounters physicians throughout the nation identify as frus-

---

Much of this introductory material is excerpted from "Empathic Communication, a teachable and learnable skill" by Platt and Keller (17).

trating. In each workshop, a number of doctors identify as "most difficult encounters" those in which the patient expresses a strong negative emotion, such as anger, sadness, or fear, or those involving a patient who seems unwilling or unable to assume responsibility for his own self-destructive behavior, such as cigarette smoking, alcoholism, or overeating.

Similar difficulties plague the doctors in training whom I have observed over the last 20 years at Presbyterian/Saint Lukes in Denver and at other hospitals throughout the country. When I first reported my observations in 1979, I called this category of physician dysfunction "The Untherapeutic Doctor" [10]. I exemplified the syndrome with a physician who left out every possible comforting gesture or action. He didn't knock on closed doors, didn't introduce himself, didn't warn the patient about painful maneuvers, and missed all the empathic opportunities. But more puzzling to me at the time were several physicians in training who seemed to do everything right— except for catching those empathic opportunities.

Patients, indeed all persons, seek to be understood. We all wish to have our feelings, ideas, concerns, and dilemmas understood. An empathic action or comment can communicate such understanding.

Patients suffer from many symptoms including pain, dyspnea, fear, and sadness. One, above all, yields to empathy: the feeling of isolation. Strong painful emotions such as anger, fear, sadness, or the paralysis of indecision are isolating. An action that breaks this isolation is strongly therapeutic.

Doctors often have difficulty doing that. Physicians report distress and lack of therapeutic tools to deal with an angry patient, a tearful patient, a frightened patient, or one who seems unable to make a pressing decision.

I believe that a route out of this difficulty is a specific interactional skill that we call an EMPATHIC ACTION. The literature offers various definitions of empathy [11–16]. What follows is the one we use in the Miles workshops and that I believe works best in resident training. It is a step-by-step process that is easily mastered and applied and that physicians report finding helpful in troublesome patient encounters [17].

1. BE AWARE OF THE AFFECTIVE MOMENT. One has to keep an ear open for statements that are full of strong feeling. Be especially attuned to strong anger, sadness, loss, grief, fear, or expressions of being trapped or stuck. Often the doctor is first aware of such an affect by paying attention to his or her own feelings. If the doctor feels frightened, angry, sad, or frustrated, it is possible that the patient feels the same way. Strong affects are contagious, but *catching* a contagious affect is not the same as the "act of feeling with the patient" that may be an end result of an empathic connection.

2. STOP AND REFLECT. Nothing is more important. Frequently the doctor has no clear idea just what strong affect has been detected. Unless the doctor takes time for reflection, it will be difficult to identify the affect. The doctor may have to stop the patient in the midst of the interview to process what has been heard.

   EXAMPLE:

   DR: Hmm. Let me stop and think about what you've been telling me for a moment.
   PT: It's just that nobody seems to be able to . . .
   DR: Please, Mr. Smith, give me a second; let me think a little. I know that you are anxious to talk about this. But I need a few moments to reflect on what you have been telling me so far.

   During this time-out, the doctor should be considering several questions, including: "How do I feel right now?" and "How is this patient feeling right now?" The thinking task isn't over until the doctor has at least one hypothesis for "How is this patient feeling right now?"
   I realize that a lot of mental processing may be taking place during this time-out. As Book [11] makes clear, one has to sort out one's own feelings, diagnose the patient's feelings, and formulate a plan. I include all this in our shorthand exhortation to "STOP."

3. NAME THE AFFECT. Sometimes the doctor will be wrong. Naming an affect requires a diagnostic guess, and as with other diagnoses, we may be wrong. If so, the patient will usually correct us.

EXAMPLE:

DR: That sounds awful. You must have been really frightened.

PT: Not so much frightened as angry. They said they would be around if I needed them, and then when I called, nobody was in.

DR: I see. Not so much frightened as angry. I can imagine how angry I would be if I had been in your shoes.

Many doctors seem to feel a great compulsion to "do something" at this point. Perhaps sensing the power of an empathic connection, they feel obliged to rush on to some sort of further action, some advice or some therapy. Part of the difficulty is the sudden surge of real feeling that we can experience when we do understand how our patients feel. We too may feel that way, and it may be painful. We come face-to-face with grief, anger, fear, and the painful realities of life and disease. Nevertheless, we believe that doctors have to learn to tolerate that swell of emotion. The power of an empathic connection is too great to squander. First we must pause in the togetherness that we have created. If the doctor's rush to move on is created by a sense that the patient cannot stand being left in such a vulnerable condition, the doctor should take heart. That patient has been all alone with the pain up to now. Our *being with* the patient will ease the pain. In fact, often we CAN do nothing more. Frequently, being together with the patient is the most therapeutic step we can provide. We must not diminish it.

4. VALIDATE THE AFFECT. Mostly this is a matter of admitting that it makes sense to feel that way. If it still doesn't make sense to you, you probably do not yet understand how the patient experiences the situation.

EXAMPLE:

DR: I can see that you were angry. But I don't exactly understand. Why angry?
PT: I had counted on them. They promised.
DR: I see. You felt betrayed.
PT: Exactly!

5. AFFIRM THE PATIENT'S PAST ACTIONS. When possible it helps to affirm the patient's past actions in order to respond to the patient's feelings. The physician may wish the patient had chosen a different course of action, but it helps to recognize that the chosen action made sense to the patient at the time the patient performed it. We are not prescribing such actions for the future, just understanding how they came to be. Our patient may have failed to follow our recommendations or missed an appointment. The patient may have become violent or attempted suicide. We don't endorse such behavior by understanding it.

6. OFFER HELP IN THE FUTURE. If possible, we can try to help in the future. If the patient gets in the same bind again, we will offer to help out. The help may be as simple as talking on the telephone or in the office.

Smith and Hoppe [18] detailed the last four of these steps. However, we are convinced that it is the first four, more than the last two, of these six steps that are critical for effective empathy. It may be that there are some native empathizers among us who never have to stop to think. For most of us, and for all of us who are troubled by affect-laden interactions, a pause to think is essential. It is this pause that identifies the empathic process as a cerebral event. As with learning any other skill, one begins in a mechanical, step-by-step fashion. Later the process becomes so smooth that it looks as if the doctor had been born to do it. "She's a natural," we say. Well, for most of us, the step-by-step approach has to be mastered first.

Consider this excerpt from a dialogue in *Conversation Failure* [19]:

PT: I keep having this pain, and nobody seems able to explain it. Dr. X and Dr. Y have done all the tests they can think of. They say that nothing turns up, and they don't know what to do next. But the pain keeps coming back.

DR: You still have the same pain?

PT: Yes. Nothing we've done has helped. Not the antacids or the Zantac or the nitroglycerin. Nothing.

DR: Well, I wouldn't be too worried. I expect that Dr. X will figure it out. He probably will have to do some more tests.

PT: [Clearly irate] What do you mean more tests? I told you. They've done everything!

This patient has just explained that he is stuck in a bad place. His doctors don't know what the cause of his pain is or what the treatment should be. This interviewing physician thought reassurance was called for. But reassurance is a dangerous tool, all too often implying that things aren't as bad as the patient thinks they are, or worse, not as bad as the patient is portraying them to be. Inappropriate and ineffective reassurance not only fails to reassure but may lead the patient to feel discounted and misunderstood. We suggest a clear message of understanding.

DR: You still have the same pain?

PT: Yes. Nothing they've done has helped. . . . Nothing.

DR: I see. You still have the pain, and your doctors are stuck. How do you feel about that?

PT: I'm a little worried.

DR: I'd be worried too, and maybe even scared.

PT: That's it, Doc. I'm really mostly frightened. I don't know whether I ought to go somewhere else or what. I think they've done everything they can, and I know they are good doctors and are trying hard. But I still have the pain.

DR: That does sound frightening. I can understand how you must feel.

Consider this sample:

PT: I felt so bad that I stopped the prednisone. I know my

kidneys get worse, but I can't help it. The other kids make fun of me for being so fat.

DR: You can't stop! The kidney disease will kill you if you don't take your medicines.

This adolescent patient had renal disease. His doctor felt immensely frustrated by the youth's decision to stop medications. She tried to convince him by explanations that verged on threats. She said that she was considering signing off the case. If the patient wouldn't follow her advice, she couldn't do anything. But we believe that she had given up too early. For one thing, the patient had returned to her. We suggested a change in posture.

DR: So you stopped the prednisone because being laughed at by the other kids was so very painful.

PT: Yes. I hated them.

DR: That must be awful. You didn't choose to be sick, and then their meanness led you to stop the only medicine that would help you. I can imagine how awful that must have felt.

PT: I knew you would be mad at me.

DR: What a trap: either the nasty remarks of your friends or an angry doctor.

PT: If I stopped the medicine.

DR: Well, I can imagine how hard that was for you, and I can even see that it seemed reasonable to stop the prednisone. But now that we've seen what happens when you stop, it makes sense to me to start it again right away. Does it to you?

PT: Yeah. I know I've got to take it.

DR: And, Sam, if you get to feeling that way again—that it would be best to stop everything—would you call me or come in and talk with me? That would help us both. It's important that we talk at times like that. I'd like to know how you're feeling and what I can do to help.

PT: I'll try, Doctor. You're not angry with me?

DR: No, Sam. I am really touched by your story. The truth is, I get really angry at those kids for being mean like that to you. And you are helping me understand how hard it is to have this kidney disease and to take these medicines we prescribe. You have to be really brave to do it.

PT: I'm not so brave.

DR: Well, I'm not sure any of us are brave all the time. I think it was brave of you, though, to come in today even though you thought I might be angry at you.

PT: I guess so.

In each case, effective empathy brings the doctor and the patient back together instead of allowing a wider rift to develop between them.

Empathy is a neologism, coined about 1910 by E. B. Titchener to serve the same function as the German word *Einfuhling*, used first in aesthetics and then by Theodor Lipps, a psychologist, to indicate a common feeling between patient and therapist [12]. *Empathy* usually has been defined as a vicarious emotion, a feeling the therapist develops from his patient, a sort of contagious affect. The usual sequence suggested is that the therapist feels a certain way, asks himself why he feels that way, and realizes that the patient has been feeling that same emotion; the affect has been transferred from one to the other. Once understood, this theory goes, contagious affect allows the therapist to act toward the patient with greater understanding.

Unfortunately, many physicians are not very aware of their own feelings. Most of us are more cognitively than emotionally aware. We may even avoid feelings, our own and others. If so, we are not likely to function well with vicarious emotion. We do much better with a cognitive approach to feelings. As our source of empathy, if we go with our strengths and think first that we have to include feelings, we will do better at counting them than if we depend on "catching" them from the patient.

It is logical to distinguish between affectively based empathy and cognitively based empathy. Grattan and Eslinger [13] define the first as "an ability to construct for oneself another's emotional experience; a sort of vicarious arousal." They define the latter as "an ability to take another's viewpoint, infer his feelings, and put yourself in his shoes." I prefer to define an empathic action in the latter sense, a cognitive skill, and view it as a learned intellectual process that requires understanding of feelings. It uses our sensory observations, what we see and hear, but then processes those observations mentally to come to a true understanding of the patient's feelings. Others call this act *self-transposal* and believe that empathy is a sort of magic feeling that may, but does not always follow. In any case, for teaching purposes and to solve the difficulties presented to us by physicians in the Miles workshops, we believe the cognitive empathic act suffices.

Doctors are often anxious about naming a strong feeling because they believe it will "put ideas in the patient's head." They suspect that telling a patient that he or she might have been frightened will, in itself, increase the patient's fear. If they name anger, they suspect that the patient will become even more angry. We doubt that such a sequence ever occurs. Our patients' strong feelings are healed by being understood and named. No patient has to have these ideas "put in his head"— most have already named them to us!

Sometimes doctors ask what to do when they are sure that a strong affect is present but are not sure just what it is. Vaughn Keller says the best rule is WHEN IN DOUBT, BE CURIOUS. It is perfectly correct to ask.

DR: I can tell that you feel strongly about this.
PT: Yes.
DR: But I am not sure I understand exactly HOW you feel. Could you tell me?

We also would apply the same rule when we recognize the feeling but not the reasons behind it. Be curious and ask. Your patient will help you out.

There are at least two patients for whom an empathic connection is insufficient or particularly difficult. The first is the patient who is angry with the very doctor who is now trying to be helpful. The second is a patient who denies the affect that seems obvious to his doctor.

If your patient is angry with you for an action that you wish you hadn't done, you may need to acknowledge your error and apologize before you can continue the dialogue.

DR: I can see how you must feel. And, as I think of it, I am truly sorry that I spoke as I did. What I said was out of line, and I have no excuse for it. I can understand your still being angry with me, but if you can forgive me, I would still like to work with you.

Or, if you don't feel so guilty, but wish to present your side of the story, you might well do so, but only after attempting an empathic action.

DR: I see. I can understand that you are really angry with me, and I can see how the matter appears to you. I would be angry too if I thought my doctor had abandoned me, as it seems to you. . . . Still, it looks different from my point of view. Would you be willing to hear how it seems to me?

The patient who denies a feeling but exemplifies that same feeling is usually very difficult to reach with an empathic effort.

DR: It sounds like you are really feeling sad about this.
PT: No, I'm not. It doesn't bother me.

Book [11] points out that it may be painful for the patient "to allow these sorts of feelings to be understood." The patient may resent feeling pitied, may feel "looked down on" or intruded upon by a sort of "mind-reading doctor." Yet there still may be hope for empathy. Even if the patient is not in touch with his or her feelings or denies possessing them, an effort to say how it might feel can be therapeutic.

DR: I see. But, you know, for many people such a terrible loss would be pretty painful. I can imagine, for example, how I'd feel. I'd feel very sad. I'd really be grieving. And I might be angry too, that it had happened to me.
PT: Yeah, I suppose so.

Many writers on the subject of empathy treat it as an innate quality that one must be born with or learn at a very early age. I disagree. I admit that the lucky physician is the one who has learned, perhaps from his or her parents, to listen to others

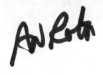

for their ideas, their feelings, and their dilemmas. But those of us who haven't been so fortunate must learn these skills if we are to function as physicians. I suspect that many physicians are specifically hampered in this area as a result of a traditional medical training that is itself abusive and unempathic. I believe that we do not teach empathy by being unempathic with our students or teach kindness by being abusive. Since communication skills are often given short shrift in medical school and residency, we are not surprised that practicing physicians not only may lack those skills but may even be unaware of their value. To a physician who has not been taught the skill, an empathic act may indeed appear like a virtuoso performance that no ordinary doctor could master.

Finally, we must consider the suspicion we all have that empathy itself is an emotion. When we understand the patient, we seem to feel for him or her, and we say just that: "I can imagine how you feel; I feel for you." I do not believe it is possible to perform the intellectual actions we are prescribing and remain distant from our patients. Even though I have described empathy as an intellectual activity, I do not believe that it is merely rational. A true understanding leads to compassion. I believe that only through understanding will we learn to feel with someone to whom we have not before felt connected. Whatever the metaphysical reality, I am convinced that an empathic action as I have defined it is a powerful tool for physicians, bridges previously great depths between doctor and patient, and can be taught and learned.

Case 7

I'M NOT TALKING

Dr. X: Hello, Mr. Y. I'm the intern on this floor, and I've come to review your history and examine you.

Y: Well you can review it in the chart. I've talked to enough doctors.

X: Pardon me?

Y: You heard me. I don't want to talk to any more doctors. It's all in the chart. What's the use of telling the same story over and over? Don't you guys talk to each other?

X: Well, yes we do. But that's why I have to go over your history, so we can discuss your case and work together.

Y: Fine, you just go out and study my chart and talk with Dr. A and Dr. B, who saw me in the emergency room. I don't need no more doctors.

X: How about if I just ask you about this illness and leave off the past history?

Y: You can leave off the whole thing. I ain't gonna talk to no more doctors. Period.

X: Are you angry with me?

Y: What would I be angry with you for? I never saw you before.

X: Well my job is to go over your history and examine you and . . .

Y: I don't care what your job is. I'm not talking.

• Now what?

This young physician felt stymied. After a little more fruitless work at persuading the patient to cooperate, he left the room and phoned the attending physician to say that he could do nothing with the patient. If the patient would not contribute a history and would not allow a physical examination, he said, there was nothing he could do.

The attending physician was distressed. He thought that the intern could have cajoled the patient into allowing at least a partial examination. He thought the intern had quit his job of data acquisition too soon. The intern thought he had suffered too long in the interchange.

• What do you consider the primary functions of the medical interview to be? If there are more than one, is there an obligatory order to pursue them?

Discussion

Of course it is true that one function of the interview is to acquire data, and if the patient won't talk, we will glean little.

However, as Julian Bird and Steve Cohen-Cole [20, 21] have told us, there are two other major functions of the interaction: building a working relationship and planning ahead. In this example, the problem is a flawed doctor-patient working relationship, and now would be a good time to attend to it. Nothing helps more to build a relationship than an effort to understand how the patient feels.

The intern could abandon trying to acquire data and try to hear what the patient is clearly telling him.

Dr. X: Uh huh. It sounds like you are fed up with telling the same story over and over to doctors who don't seem to talk with each other.

Y: Right!

X: I can see how aggravated you would be. You must wonder what use it is to tell any of us what's going on.

Y: It don't seem to do any good.

X: Like you're just spinning your wheels.

Y: In the mud.

X: Yeah. OK, I see how annoying that would be.

Y: You got it, Doc. I don't have anything against you. At least you can see how I feel.

X: OK. What can we do now? What if I go get your chart and tell you what I can learn from it. Then maybe you could fill in the blanks and correct anything I misunderstand.

Y: Yeah. I could do that.

X: You know, one of the problems is that some of the doctors dictate their notes and then the dictation isn't transcribed for 24 hours. So we might find only very abbreviated notes in the chart so far.

Y: That's OK, Doc. I'll help you fill in the blanks.

Is it hard to believe that simple empathy could do so much? Only if you are unfamiliar with this powerful tool. And of course, the physician has to act. Once we understand the patient's feeling state, we can more easily see a path of action.

Empathy is not a trick. We are not trying to trick the patient into cooperating, but once we understand his feeling state, we can more easily see our best route forward. The primary function of empathy seems to me to bring the patient and the doctor together, close enough together to let their relationship do its job.

Case 8

THINK POSITIVELY

The doctor entered his patient's hospital room and addressed the woman lying in the hospital bed. He disregarded the presence of a younger woman who was seated at the side of the bed.

Dr. P: Hello, Ms. R. I'm Dr. P. What brings you today? Why are you in the hospital?

R: Trouble breathing, I guess. Or what was it? [Turning to her daughter] Just that morning.

Daughter: She don't remember, so we don't know.

P: Well then, any other problems? Can you describe the trouble?

R: I don't remember.

D: She's diabetic.

P: You take shots?

D: She has heart trouble.

P: Any other medicines?

D: She takes Lanoxin, Lasix, Ismelin, and insulin.

P: How are you feeling now?

R: Pretty good.

P: Ready to go for a jog?

R: Yes.

P: How long have you been here in the hospital?

D: She came in four days ago. We took her to Aurora Presbyterian, and then they sent her to Denver Pres. She had a lot of cough and was short of wind and had maybe some pain.

P: How many children do you have?

R: Eight.

P: And how is your husband?

R: He died two years ago.

P: I see. And how are you coping?

R: Not too good.
P: Difficult?
D: She doesn't remember too good. It's getting worse.
P: Well, I think it is a good idea to think positively; to think about what we do have. Your daughter here is obviously very concerned about you.

- What is the key conversation problem Dr. P is facing here?
- What is the key problem the patient is having?
- What do you think about Dr. P's last comment?

Discussion

There is an old pilot adage that I like: "The landing is all in the approach." If the plane is lined up with the runway, the landing is likely to go well. If the approach is slipshod, so will the landing be. I think this adage holds for interviews too: The interview is all in the approach.

Dr. P should spend a moment or two appraising the environment before he starts his interviews. If there is another person present, he should learn that person's name and role in the patient's life. In this conversation, Dr. P failed to identify the patient's daughter and had no clear idea throughout the conversation whom he was talking with. Nor could he make sense of this strange three-pointed interaction because he didn't understand the part one of the speakers played.

His key conversation problem was the triangle, with one angle unidentified but essential for data gathering.

Mrs. R is confused. Whatever brought her to the hospital, cardiac or pulmonary symptoms, she is really most troubled by her missing memory. She and her daughter have mentioned this problem several times, and it behooves Dr. P to attend to it. He, wishing he could focus on the presumed cardiac problem, tends to ignore the mental difficulty. Too bad, since Mrs. R can't tell him much about her now absent dyspnea, but can help him to understand the level of her confusion. Then he needs to do a mental status examination.

Finally, consider that amazing little bit of "feel

good therapy," "Well I think it is a good idea to think positively. . . ." What is called for is an empathic understanding of the patient's feelings. We don't even know what they are yet, except that it has been hard to cope with the loss of her memory and her husband. The doctor could just repeat her statement: "I can imagine. It must be hard to cope." Then he could ask to be told more. I cannot see any need to rush in with an exhortation to "look on the bright side." In fact, such an exhortation tends to discount the patient's perspective and could only lead her to feel undervalued and unheard.

It seems that we can't solve this patient's emotional state without understanding our own. I'd suggest that Dr. P stop when Mrs. R mentions her feelings of bereavement and ask himself how he is feeling. Is he feeling sad? Angry? Unsure how to proceed? Frightened? Does he think he has done his patient damage by opening up a sore area? Until the doctor understands his own feelings he is unlikely to be able to help his patient with hers. Once the doctor acknowledges his own feelings, he might then be able to ask himself or perhaps ask his patient how she might be feeling to have said what she said. I like that sequence. It reminds me of the theme of C. S. Lewis's *Till We Have Faces* [22]: How can we see others until we can see ourselves?

Dr. P said that he feared opening up a "Pandora's box" of strong feelings, perhaps of overwhelming sadness. But the sadness is there and has already been let out of the box. Now the challenge is to GET WITH the patient, to diminish the isolation that sadness imposes. It's one thing to feel sad. It's worse to name the sadness and then be left alone with it.

And what if you have missed the golden opportunity to consider your own and then your patient's feelings? What if you have already blurted out an exhortation to cheerfulness? I think there is always time to reconsider.

Dr. P: Oh gosh! Let me stop for a moment. I want to rethink this.

R: It's all right, Doctor, I don't think it matters.

P: No, I really want to stop to think. Let me just be silent and mull for a moment.

[Silence.]

P: OK, I think I understand. You were telling me that it has
   been really hard since your husband died.
R: We were together for 45 years.
P: I can imagine. It must be really tough.
R: It is, Doctor. My kids help out, of course.
P: But you still miss him.
R: Yes.

I think the key to the concept of conversation repair is that
it is possible to establish a good relationship even if we have
begun it badly. If we are sincere and keep our eyes open, we
can catch our errors and repair them. After all, any carpenter
can do a good job the first time. It takes a master carpenter to
make mistakes and then figure out how to fix them.

Case 9

IT'S NOT THE RIGHT TIME

W: I see that my cholesterol is sky high.
Dr. F: That's right, it seems to be increasing.
W: And my HDL isn't going up despite exercise.
F: No.
W: And you told me that the LDL is really worse, and now it's
   over 200.
F: True.
W: This is really stupid! I know what to do, but I just can't
   leave those desserts alone. I eat every one they put in front
   of me. And ice cream too.
F: Well, Bill, we really aren't so sure how much to worry about
   these numbers in a 70-year-old man who doesn't smoke,
   has no worrisome family history, and most important,
   hasn't had any heart disorder so far. Most of our studies
   have been done in younger men. If we're worried about
   premature heart disease, you can't really get that, not at
   age 70. Still, any heart attack would be premature as far as
   you or I are concerned.

W: That's right. Just because I'm 70 is no reason I need a heart attack. I've got to do something about this cholesterol.

F: OK. Well, we could do one of three things. We could leave it alone.

W: The French say that if a thing isn't absolutely necessary that it be done, then it is absolutely necessary that we not do it.

F: OK. Or you could make a real effort to avoid all fats for two or three weeks and repeat the lipid levels. Or we could start you on a cholesterol-lowering agent like lovastatin.

W: I think I'd really like to try to change my eating. Wouldn't that be logical?

F: Yes, I think so. To avoid fats, you have to avoid butter and margarine . . .

W: Margarine too? Mine says it is low fat.

F: That means it is more water or air, but you probably defeat that by using more of it.

W: I do. Yes, true, I do.

F: And avoid oils, salad dressings, milk fat, ice cream, almost any sweets except hard candies, avoid fried foods, fatty meats, cheese, nuts . . .

W: I'm beginning to doubt that this could be done with my schedule. I travel a lot, and I eat out a lot.

[Pause.]

W: It's not that I don't think I should do it, even could do it. It's just that this is not the right time. It's not the right time.

F: Not the right time?

W: I guess it never is the right time.

F: For this or for lots of other things. Do you remember Peter Seller's refrain in the Pink Panther movies? "Now is not the time, Kato!"

W: Well, maybe we need to go with plan B.

- How does one know when is the right time to act?

- What do you call the skill of putting off for tomorrow what doesn't absolutely have to be done today?

Discussion

We are all expert at procrastination, but there are few rules about when to act.

The people who have done the most writing about decision points in behavioral disorders are the alcohol treatment people. They speak of "hitting bottom." Drinkers who decide to abstain often can recognize a specific point of decision, often associated with some worsening of their usual behavior or its outcomes beyond a point they can tolerate anymore. For one alcoholic, being arrested for driving under the influence might be that decision point. For another, injuring an innocent person in an automobile accident might be the event that tells the drinker to stop. Perpetrators of behavioral disorders such as cigarette smoking, drug abuse, domestic violence, or shoplifting have identified similar catalysts for change. Hitting bottom is less often mentioned in connection with therapy for eating disorders, perhaps because the change involves a different degree of abstention from the behavior.

What can we do to help W with his decision? This doctor seemed content to accept the fact that now was not the time. A better strategy might be to help the patient understand that you understand his ambivalence and the dilemma he is in, an attempt at empathy.

F: It seems that you are caught in a dilemma.
W: What do you mean?
F: Well, it seems to me that you understand full well the adverse effects of continuing as you are now. You know that you are risking your very life. But you enjoy eating, enjoy your lifestyle with the traveling and the good food.
W: Absolutely. I love those desserts.
F: So you are caught between two conflicting desires.
W: Yes.
F: How are you going to resolve the conflict?
W: Hmm. I guess I have to think more about it.

By the way, we might pause for a moment to reaffirm how

critical it is for a physician to be able to do what is needed now, right now! I think the ability to act now, to do what is needed without putting it off past the critical moment, is a vital personality feature needed to practice medicine.

Of course, it may be helpful to know that this patient at this time cannot carry out plan A! We don't have to go through the frustration of trying to convince him to do it, then watch the process fail. We don't have to feel unsuccessful if he can look at the task and say he cannot do it. For this patient, normally a very decisive person with great responsibilities, a better course was perhaps to use the lipid-lowering agent and not to insist on major dietary changes just now. It seemed so to him and thus probably was.

Case 10

CHOKING TO DEATH

The patient was a 60-year-old retired journalist. Because his physician had also recently retired, Mr. B called a new doctor, Dr. S, during an episode of marked dyspnea. Hospitalized, he failed to improve but continued down a very short hill, to die in the hospital a month after admission. His diagnosis: cigarettism with resultant chronic obstructive lung disease.

During his hospital stay, the doctor had this discussion with his new patient.

Dr. S: How do you feel about the smoking?
B: Well, I [pause to breathe] don't feel [pause to breathe] guilty.
S: That's good. What do you mean?
B: No one [pause] told me.
S: Really? That's hard to believe. Dr. X would surely have told you.
B: That's true. [Pause] He said that if I didn't stop, [pause] I'd have trouble. So I figured I'd wait [pause] until then to stop. Nobody told me I'd [pause] spend the last two years choking to death.
S: Ah! I see. Nobody told you that you would spend your last years choking to death.

B: That's right. You doctors ought [pause] to tell your patients that they will choke [pause] to death. Then I would have [pause] stopped smoking. Maybe.

- Should we tell our patients that they will choke to death?
- How might we do that?
- How can we improve our success at getting smokers to desist?

Discussion

What can we do for our cigarette-smoking patients? I've tried all sorts of ploys; the venal:

P: I think it's a good idea for you to smoke. I still have two daughters in college, and I like to take vacations to Europe. So I need you to continue smoking. That makes a lot of business for me.

or the prophetic:

P: Cigarette smoking is the toughest addiction to break. But you have your fate in your own hands. What you do about smoking will influence your future health to a greater degree than any other act of yours or of mine.

After hearing this interchange between Dr. S and Mr. B, I incorporated a choking-to-death demonstration. I asked my patients to close one nostril and breathe through only the narrower one. While they sat quietly, focusing on the next breath, I told them that their last two years will be spent looking for the next breath. I recounted Mr. B's story and told them that the last two years would be spent choking to death. Try it yourself! It is an impressive exercise. But, does it work? Maybe a little, just as most of our efforts to help patients stop smoking help a little.

According to experts, you can do the following:

1. Be sure your office is a nonsmoking place.

2. Be sure you ask about smoking at every visit; note the number of daily cigarettes.

3. Be sure you advise your patient about smoking at each visit.

4. Include the diagnosis "disease of tobacco use," code #305.11. I call it CIGARETTISM.

5. Do what you can politically to discourage cigarette use and sales in your community. When they are willing, refer your patients to smoke-ending programs.

G. C. Williams et al. [23] suggest asking the following three questions:

1. What is your understanding of the relationship between smoking and your health?

2. Are you considering or ready to quit smoking?

3. What can we do to help you reach this decision?

I believe that the best and most therapeutic posture we can use is that of empathy. If we understand our patients better and they know that we do understand, we have made a connection that may let us be influential in their lifestyle choices. Empathy here is mostly a matter of empathizing with the patient's occult dilemma, with the fix he is in.

Dr. S: I can see that you are caught in a difficult dilemma. On one hand, you can see that the smoking is bad for your health. You tell me about your cough and your breathing trouble, and you know that smoking causes lung cancer, heart disease, and emphysema. On the other hand, you enjoy smoking, find that it calms you and helps you focus your mind, and you found it distressing in the past when you tried to quit.

B: That's right, Doc.

S: So you are really caught between a rock and a hard place. How are you going to resolve the dilemma? What are you going to do?

Such an empathic posture will probably be more helpful to our patients than my guerilla tactics. Scare tactics rarely work for people who are addicted to any drug, but an empathic approach coupled with supportive statements to say that you will be there to help your patients quit whenever they are ready is more effective and more humane.

Case 11

WHAT'S MY HEMOGLOBIN

Mr. X (a middle-aged man, an accountant, who pulls out a large pocket notebook as he sits down in the examining room chair): Hello, Doctor.

Dr. Y: Hello, Mr. X. It's nice to see you. How do you feel?

X: I don't know yet. Let's see. [Reading from notebook] Friday, November 12, 47.1 on hematocrit. This was . . . umm . . . gastrointestinal clinic.

Y: November 12th?

X: Yeah, November 12. About a month before, I was up on the ninth floor to look everything over. OK, this was the final thing, he told me in five years they might reappear. Perfect! Five days later I'm bleeding again. Then I saw you Wednesday, November 17, five days later, 45.9.

Y: Right.

X: OK, that's when you gave me suppositories. Then I saw you the following Wednesday, [checks notebook again] November 24. It stopped; we had a miracle.

Y: Good!

X: Well otherwise I wondered why I bled anyway, but I'll ask you that later. [Writes in notebook.] Then, that Saturday, which was December 4, I saw my friend in his apartment at 6:30. I started to bleed like mad.

Y: How much blood?

X: A lot. Just like upstairs at the hospital.

Y: Filling up the toilet bowl?

X: Oh yeah, lots. OK. [Reads again from notebook] Car accident Saturday, vacation starts Monday. I've got written out I was bleeding all the way to the middle of January. Do you have my hemoglobin? Is it back today? What's my hemoglobin? [Writes in notebook.]

Y: Oh. Well, why don't you backtrack first. Tell me what has happened from the fourth of January when you stopped bleeding . . .

X: The middle of January.

Y: The middle of January, up to now in March.

X: [Appears to be angry] Well, I'm telling you, everything's happened.

Y: OK.

X: I was in terrible shape. I was out of suppositories; I went to get some more . . .

Y: How much bleeding in the last month?

X: Well, I'm not bleeding.

Y: You're not bleeding any more?

X: Well, I checked my thing, and my hemoglobin was 41.

Y: Your hematocrit.

X: No, not hematocrit. Hemoglobin! They call it the red blood.

Y: OK, yeah, when did they check that and find it was 41?

X: Monday.

Y: Where did you go?

X: I went to the clinic my friend works at. All I went for was to see what my protein was. My protein was high, 7.4.

- What is all this concern for laboratory detail?
- Should the physician explain more about the difference between hematocrit and hemoglobin?

Discussion

Why does this patient talk about laboratory tests when we would prefer him to tell us his symptoms? This doctor thought his patient's data to be unimportant and wished to hear more symptoms and less "doctor talk." Perhaps this patient is trying to imitate the doctors he consults who seem so often to focus on blood tests or x-rays as precise indicators of disease or cure. And of course, if the laboratory data are relatively unimportant, it is even less important to belabor the difference between hemoglobin and hematocrit.

Probably this patient reduces anxiety by being in control of data. His notebook is a tidy way of containing his life. We might try to approach his basic anxiety. It would be fair to ask how worried he was about this recurrent bleeding.

Y: That sounds pretty scary to have so much bleeding with so little warning.
X: You aren't kidding, Doc. And it doesn't help for the surgeon to tell me I'm gonna be OK for five years, and then it starts to bleed again in five days.
Y: I can imagine how frightening and how frustrating it must be for you. I imagine that you probably feel unable to control this trouble.
X: I don't like that feeling, Doc.
Y: No. You usually are pretty much in control of your world; this bleeding trouble is pretty frustrating.
X: It sure is. I wish I had a better way to deal with it.
Y: Well, let's talk about it. Would you like some suggestions?

Is this a likely outcome? I think an empathic route usually gets results. Stephen Cohen-Cole [21] says, "When in doubt we should attempt to empathize with the patient." But Dr. Y tells me that empathy didn't work with this patient, who, he says, is "not in touch with his feelings." He responds to an empathic response with a blank stare and more attention to his notebook and hemoglobin values.

We shouldn't be too surprised that psychopathology can overcome an empathic technique. This patient may be too obsessive to let us near his underlying anxiety. Perhaps the best we can do is to get him to keep track of symptoms instead of laboratory values. Then we will run the risk of hearing an endless and carefully recorded litany of each and every cramp, belch, and flatus.

We can also consider extending the system with a psychiatric consultation. We really have as yet no understanding of what is driving the patient to such obsessive behavior. If we can't find out, perhaps one of our more psychologically trained colleagues can.

I JUST WANT TO CONSULT WITH THE DOCTOR

Ms. R appeared as a new patient at Dr. X's office but refused to have her vital signs measured by the doctor's assistant. "I don't want an examination," she said. "I just want to consult with the doctor." When he entered the room, their conversation began:

X: Hello, you must be Ms. R. I'm Dr. X. I'm glad to meet you.

R: Hello, Doctor. I'm not sure that I'm in the right place. I lost my regular doctor when my husband's company changed insurance. Then I got another doctor. And, oh me, it's a long story.

X: That's hard—to lose a doctor you like because of a change in insurance.

R: Yes, and then I went to Dr. B. But I got sick with some bronchitis, and she treated me with two grams a day of an antibiotic. I got itchy and sick, and I went back, but Dr. B couldn't see me. So I saw her associate, Dr. C. He said, "That's the wrong antibiotic for you." And he put me on some other pills. So I thought I shouldn't see Dr. B any more. I didn't think she had treated me right, and then she couldn't see me when I was worse.

X: I see.

R: Yes, and I thought I ought to have a woman doctor, so I found Dr. D, and she examined me, but she left off the Pap smear, and she didn't do a rectal examination even though I told her about my bleeding hemorrhoids. Then she checked my blood sugar, and it was high, so she said I needed insulin.

X: Uh huh?

R: And I asked for a second opinion, and she said she couldn't do that or the insurance would penalize her. I was upset, and I didn't think I should start insulin so quickly.

X: Yes? And then?

R: Well, I called Washington National Insurance, and they said I had several options and one was to change primary doctors, and they suggested you.

X: I see. What about your concern to have a female doctor?

R: Well, I thought that maybe I would be going into the meno-
pause soon. I'm 43, and I had a period come early last week.
And I thought maybe a woman doctor would be best for
me. But now I've had two female doctors in a row, and I
don't know anymore.

- Are you filled with dread by this doctor-shopper?
- Do you have your list of local female physicians handy?
  Do you know which of them participates with Washington
  National Insurance?

Discussion

This sequence of events may be a warning. But forewarned is
forearmed. Her tale of difficulties with past physicians is a gift
to you. Now you know more about what to do to satisfy her
needs, and you have a lot of her distress out in the open.

You might start with a clear statement of recognition of the
difficulties she's gone through. In fact, that's just what this
doctor did.

X: What a difficult time you've had! You had to try several
doctors, and you still don't know if you have the right one.
You thought perhaps a female physician would be best, and
then you were dissatisfied with two, one for the bad experience you had when she treated you with an antibiotic and
the other for her lack of thoroughness and the feeling you
had that you were being rushed into insulin therapy.

R: That's right, doctor. And I'm really frightened too. My body
seems to be going bad on me. I've had high blood pressure
for a long time, and it seemed to be doing OK, but when I
heard that I had diabetes, my blood pressure was up too.

X: I see. It seems that you are falling apart at the young age of
43. How are things going at home?

R: Pretty good. My husband wants me to take care of my health,
and he keeps telling me to get to the doctor. But he doesn't
give me the support I'd like.

X: The support you'd like?

R: Yes. I'd like him to come to the doctor with me, and he doesn't want to.

X: I see. So you're unsure just who can help you medically and how, a little distressed that your husband wants you to get well but won't come along to the doctor, and afraid that your health is going downhill.

R: That's true.

X: Well, I think we could work together if you wanted. Or, if you are sure you need a woman doctor, I would be glad to recommend one who is in your insurance group. If we did work together though, I have a request to make. If we have difficulties or if something I do is unsatisfactory, I would like you to talk with me about it before going off to another doctor.

R: That seems quite reasonable, Doctor. And I think we could work together, too.

X: OK. In that case, let me review your medical history now, and we will schedule you back soon to do a good examination. And in the meantime we will gather some information about your sugars and what you are eating. How's that?

R: That sounds just right. Thank you, Doctor. They told me at Washington National that they would send me to the best they had. I think they did.

Do you wonder how things will go at the next visit? Do you speculate that she will tell you that she has just found an endocrinologist who altered your protocols? In fact this patient was content with Dr. X's approach, did remain with him, and did quite well in further caring for her diabetes.

Case 13

THORACIC OUTLET SYNDROME

Dr. A: Well, Ms. Rigor, what sort of trouble brings you to me?

R: The biggest trouble, Doctor, is that I can't find anyone who really understands my thoracic outlet syndrome. No one can understand how much trouble it causes me.

A: I see. What sort of symptoms does it cause?

R: I can't do anything with my arms. I am totally disabled from this, and no one understands. One doctor after another has failed me.

A: Uh huh?

R: My friend, Sheila, has this trouble too. She was the one who told me what was wrong with me. No doctor had been able to diagnose it.

A: And the symptoms are?

R: I told you! I have thoracic outlet syndrome. I shouldn't have to tell you what that is. You're supposed to know.

A: Well, you know, we doctors like to hear symptoms instead of diagnoses. We do better then.

R: Pain! I have pain all over in my arms and my hands. I can't do anything with them. I can't write or type. I almost can't feed myself.

A: And you've had nerve conduction studies?

R: No, I haven't. I'm not going to allow anyone to cause me more pain. It's already as severe as I can stand. Besides, the doctors almost ruined my friend with needles and tests. I won't let you do that to me.

A: What other troubles have you had?

R: Mostly doctors. My mother's doctors misdiagnosed her too. They caused her so much pain that I had to quit work to care for her. If I hadn't come home to care for her, she would have died right then.

A: And besides that?

R: I've got everything. I've had hypertension since I was 22. My ankles swell up; they've done it since 1970. My triglycerides are too high, and my cholesterol is too. I have a metabolic abnormality. Then my arms started swelling in 1990. I need to take Maxzide and Percodan, and I need refills on my Pamelor too.

A: You've had arm trouble for a long time then?

R: No, Doctor, I told you, it started after my accident in 1991. I was closing a window and it wasn't well anchored, and it came down on my hand.

A: All right. Suppose we stop now and do an examination . . .

R: Oh, you can't do that, Doctor. I can't permit you to examine me. It hurts too much. If you tapped my arm with a reflex hammer, my arm would swell for a month and I'd have terrible pain.

A: How am I to come to any diagnoses if I can't examine you?

R: I told you. I have thoracic outlet syndrome. I just need more pain medicine.

- What can we do when the patient refuses to cooperate with our usual procedure, for example, to allow a physical examination?
- What do you think happened here?
- Any way out of the trouble?
- This case was presented to a group of physicians at a workshop at the 1993 Annual American College of Physicians Meeting. They all agreed that this case was hopeless. What do you think?

Discussion

What happened here? This doctor despaired of doing anything useful with this patient. He told her:

A: I don't think I'm going to be able to properly diagnose and treat you without being able to complete a physical examination. Therefore, I won't charge you for today's visit. I don't think I'll be able to take care of you.

He escorted the patient to the front desk and bid her adieu.

Standing at the appointment counter, she began to pound her fists and arms on the counter and scream. Her screams were inarticulate "aaah, aaah" sounds. She left the office screaming and carried on in the same way outside the door and down the walkway. Other patients in the office looked up and asked, "Is there something out there in pain? Some sort of an animal?" The office staff were amazed. The doctor was distressed and felt his interaction with this patient had been a failure but saw no way he could have done better.

What might have been done? Boy, this is a tough one! Recall Cohen-Cole's [21] concept of three main tasks in our communication with patients: data gathering, relationship building, and planning ahead. We often act as if our sole interest, or at least our first task, is data gathering. Perhaps we'd do better to be more flexible. In this case I wonder if the doctor might have recognized earlier on that he was going to have difficulty gathering data and that there were major relationship problems that needed attention first. For example, right at the beginning when the patient says that she is having trouble getting doctors to understand, he could have said:

A: You feel pretty misunderstood then by most doctors.

And after "One doctor after another has failed me," he could try:

A: It sounds pretty hard for you. You haven't been able to get what you need from your doctors.

Or consider her comments about her mother. He might try:

A: It sounds like you've had trouble with other doctors.
R: They didn't diagnose her right.
A: And that makes it harder for you to trust doctors and their diagnostic abilities.
R: Yeah.

None of these interjections have much to do with data gathering, but all, in their empathic function, improve relationships and might lead to the possibility of working together.

Greg Carroll and Vaughn Keller of the Miles Institute for Health Care Communication say that when matters are deteriorating, we should stop to examine our own feelings. I asked Dr. A how he was feeling as this interview progressed. He said that he wasn't angry. He admitted that he felt sad and hopeless. He couldn't see any way he would "win" in this encounter. And he felt trapped. I was surprised to hear a denial of anger, since I perceive this patient to be angry and think her anger would quickly cathect my own if I were the doctor. But Dr. A probably has a higher threshold for anger than I do.

Once the doctor has sorted out his own feelings, he has a choice. Should he let the patient in on how he is feeling? Sometimes it helps, but it is not obligatory. He might give her a hint.

A: Ms. R, I am having some difficulty. I am beginning to wonder if I will be able to help you. I feel caught between what you expect and what I think I have to do to be a good doctor.
R: What do you mean?
A: Well, I usually feel obliged to examine my patients to satisfy myself about the diagnosis before prescribing anything, and I can hear you say that you are afraid that an examination might be too painful for you.
R: I'm sure it would.
A: So that makes it hard for me to do my job. How do you think we should proceed?

Perhaps then they could negotiate some arrangement. Perhaps, for example, Dr. A could offer to give her a week's worth of the medications she seeks and then to see her back in the office with plans to do a complete examination in seven days. He could ask her to consider the matter; if she still found it impossible, she could use the week to find another doctor.

If the doctor is willing to work with this patient, he has to decide where to start. Dr. Jane Lee says that she would start with whatever is making it hard for her to trust doctors. Why is she afraid of doctors? What has happened to HER in the hands of doctors? What precisely happened to her friend? What is she fearful of? And there are other puzzles: Why does she continue to consult doctors if all have failed her? Why not try naturopathy, a chiropractor, massage therapy, acupuncture, dietary supplements, Christian Science, or meditation? Is it just that she wants or needs the drugs that only an allopath can prescribe?

Finally, we might consider the diagnosis. Is this woman psychotic? It is often impossible to deal rationally with someone who is psychotic. Or does she fit in one of the diagnostic groupings that often seem the result of prolonged childhood sexual or physical abuse? Borderline personality disorder, multiple personalities, and somatization disorder patients often have such histories. Doctors often have great difficulty dealing with such patients, often use pejorative labels, and often fear and dislike their interactions with these people. Judith Herman [24] describes the tasks of the therapist quite clearly. We need to work toward uncovering the underlying trauma and empathically witnessing for the patient. Such a task is not likely to be accomplished in the first interview, but we do best if we achieve some sort of working relationship with the patient, with plans to explore for long-term psychopathology later. Is this reasonable for an internist? I think so, since we are usually the doctors to whom these patients come.

Case 14

HYPERBOLE, INDEED

During rounds with attending physicians, an intern described a difficult patient who hadn't wanted to talk to him on admission. The patient had insisted that "it was all in the chart" and that he had "already talked to too many doctors; he wasn't going to talk to another."

The attending physician commiserated with the intern. "He had been a difficult patient," he agreed. Then he suggested that using hyperbole may help one deal with such patients. Sometimes it helps to let patients know that you have really heard them if you exaggerate what they say. You might try something like this: "Well, here I am, the twentieth doctor you've seen today." Of course you are using hyperbole as evidence of your understanding of his distress, a sort of empathic comment.

The intern agreed that the technique might be useful and that he might try it someday. Ten days later the same intern approached the same attending physician and said that he had tried the hyperbole technique, but that it had backfired. He had a patient who was depressed, glum, hostile, and uncooperative. The patient kept his room dark, the shades and curtains pulled, the lights dimmed. The patient usually was uncooperative and unfriendly. This morning, trying out the new technique, the dialogue had gone this way:

Dr. X: [In a very loud and cheery voice] Well, good morning! Let me just pull open your curtains here! [which he did, quite vigorously.] What a great day! This is the kind of day to really enjoy!

Mr. Y: What the hell! Get the hell out of here! Get out! Get out and don't come back!

- What went wrong?
- Why didn't hyperbole work here?

Discussion

Of course, the job is to let your patient know that you really understand how he feels. Empathic "getting with the patient" decreases the distance between you and lessens the patient's isolation. Usually we are best off using simple declarative statements like "I can see that you are really feeling glum. It looks as if you can hardly even stand to let the day into your room. That looks really painful."

But life would be dull if we couldn't exercise our inventiveness and occasionally use jests, exaggeration, and even outrageous comments. To be sure, these devices must be used very precisely. Hyperbole, for instance, must be a matter of exaggerating the patient's feelings, not the doctor's. If one is to exaggerate, it is the patient's feelings, not the doctor's, that have to be attended to. The doctor might have tried this approach:

X: It's pretty dark in here. This must be the cave of someone who is pretty glum. No sun would ever shine here. No sun, no cheer, no hope. Nope, this is not a cheerful room today.

Y: You got it, doc. That's exactly how I feel.

X: I can see that. Just being in here makes me feel sad. I think I'll just lie down on the floor. I don't think I can go on with my life.

Y: Come on, Doc. I'm the one who's depressed. Besides, I don't feel quite that bad today.

X: Oh? Well, then, perhaps I can crack the shades a little, let a
   tiny ray of light in on us.
Y: Yeah, why don't you do that. I can stand it.

See? Again, the point of the hyperbole technique is to exaggerate the patient's feelings, in this case sadness and hope-
lessness, not the doctor's cheery state.

3

Acknowledgment

How can I listen to her when little Johnny, age two, is dismantling my office?

Dr. Xylom

Till that word can be dug out of us, why should the gods hear the babble that we think we mean? How can they meet us face to face till we have faces?

C. S. Lewis [22]

When physician-patient encounters go wrong, we're half the trouble. Can we ever believe that? If you review the literature of troubled doctor-patient interactions, as White and Keller [25] have done, you will find that most of the articles in medical journals blame the patient. We talk about "The Hateful Patient," "The Difficult Patient," and so on. You won't come up with much looking for articles about the difficult doctor. But surely in any interaction, both parties bear scrutiny.

In a medical interaction, then, we can expect to find that the doctor's feelings and actions lead to difficulty half the time, but we expect the doctor to find and fix the problem all the time. If I am the cause of the trouble and I am still saddled with the need to analyze it, sort it out, and remedy it, I have a terrific burden. It may be too much. Unfortunately, even if they have a high level of self-confidence, most patients are too handicapped by the great power imbalance in the doctor-patient interaction to ask for what they need, to confront the doctor, and to take charge of the medical encounter. We can't expect them to do it. We have to do it ourselves.

How to go about it? I suggest a process of acknowledgment. The first step, as always when things are going wrong, is to be aware that something is going wrong. The next step is to think about it. Consider your own feelings. How are you feeling? Is it one of the bad old feelings that you have known since child-hood? Something specific to your personality? An individual response? If so, what do you need to do to get your response under control? Do you need to take time out? Even excuse yourself from the room for a few minutes? Do you want to share your difficulty with your patient? Maybe yes, maybe no, but it's your decision.

Perhaps you've identified that the difficulty resides in the patient. You usually need to talk to him about it. You should follow good communication techniques: Speak for yourself, from the "I position," claiming the problem as your own, and asking for help from the patient. Sometimes the patient will deny the problem, but usually not if you are neither blaming nor humiliating him.

Consider this little conversation, for example:

Patient Y: I'm um uh sshylly nl sthan n.

Dr. X: [To himself] Why doesn't this man speak up? He mumbles in his beard, and I can't understand what he's saying. I don't know why I always get saddled with such people. They must pick me out. I'M HAVING DIFFICULTY HERE.

X: [Aloud] Mr. Y, I'm having a little difficulty.

Y: Ths era. Is prly y trl. Ern s.

X: No, really, Mr. Y. Please don't talk for a minute. I need to stop to think.

X: [To himself] I really feel angry. What am I angry about? He's inarticulate, is that it? Do I feel unappreciated because he hasn't been able to speak clearly? Personally offended? No? Well, maybe I can stop feeling angry. In fact, I feel better already. I think I can share it with him.

X: [Aloud] Mr. Y, I'm having a hard time hearing you distinctly.

I think it would help if we turn off the television here [does so], and I wonder if there is anything you can do to help me.

Y: I cd spou th gm.

X: Spit out the gum?

Y: Ye.

X: OK, how about trying that. Then I will pull up my chair closer and perhaps you could try to speak a little bit louder too. Would you be able to do that?

Y: [Now gumless] Yeah.

That's better than blaming the patient and perhaps getting in an argument with him.

More difficult situations involve very strong feelings on the part of the doctor. Feelings of anger, fear, sadness, entrapment, or being discounted may trigger reactions of fleeing or fighting. Amorous feelings may trigger actions that will destroy the doctor-patient relationship. We need to stop, think about our feelings, consider their sources (often not just the patient who is with us right now), and decide how to proceed. Disregarding our own strong feelings is perilous; we should not do that.

Remember Case 2, "I'm Really Upset"? How much more effective Dr. X would have been if he had consulted his own feelings, discussed his bewilderment with the patient, and asked for her help!

What sort of troubles hamper doctors? Remember the frustration exercise in the Miles Physician-Patient Communication workshops? Physicians are asked to name and describe the doctor-patient interactions that they find most difficult. The lists generated by different groups are remarkably similar. Here is a typical list:

1. Patient brings a laundry list of problems.
2. Theorist—patient gives theories rather than symptoms.
3. "By the way"—most important problem surfaces at the end of interview.
4. Patient has his or her own diagnosis and wants to convince the doctor of it.

5. "My chiropractor says"—patient brings suggestions from other care-takers, usually those the doctor distrusts.

6. Patient comes with plan in mind, perhaps drug seeking.

7. Patient doesn't follow doctor's instructions, then blames him or her for bad outcome.

8. Narrator rambles.

9. Patient is aphasic.

10. Patient does not speak English well.

11. Patient abuses doctor's office staff but treats doctor very politely.

12. Patient is determined not to be helped. "Nothing has ever helped me and nothing ever will."

13. Insurance company won't allow referral and patient wants one.

14. Patient calls Friday at 4 P.M. with a problem that has been present for two weeks.

15. Patient brings wild child who tears apart doctor's examining room while the doctor tries to attend to mother's medical needs.

16. Mother brings one child to be seen but then asks doctor to attend to her three other children whom she has also brought in.

17. Patient wants telephone prescription.

18. Emergency call. When doctor calls back promptly, the patient is out and the doctor has to talk to an answering machine.

19. Compensation case. Accident victim who won't get well.

20. Malingerer.

21. Insurance company badgers doctor about admissions.

22. Ambulance kidnaps patient to another hospital where doctor doesn't have privileges.

23. Child is brought to doctor by babysitter; then doctor has to call and talk to three different family members.

24. Patient doesn't follow doctor's recommendations, even when he or she writes them out.

25. Cigarette smoker wants cure for his chronic bronchitis.
26. Alcoholic won't take responsibility for his or her behavior.
27. Noninformative—patient willing to talk but seems not to understand his or her own symptoms.
28. Doctor is backed up, and patient needs more time.
29. Patient whines.
30. Patient is angry, threatening, or obnoxious.
31. Parent insists on specific therapy for the child, perhaps the most expensive therapy.
32. Patient seems to agree with everything doctor says but is unconvinced and then does not comply.
33. Depressed, somatizing patient refuses psychotherapy.
34. Passive patient won't take responsibility.
35. Patient with a chronic illness who is making no therapeutic progress demands more from doctor.
36. VIP patient who is arrogant.
37. Spouse tells the story.
38. Patient gives different story to different interviewers.
39. Patient won't talk to doctor. "It's all in my chart."

Many of these frustrating experiences can be approached with acknowledgment of the problem and enlistment of the patient. Surely these would yield to such an approach:

1. Laundry list, multiple complaints.
2. Noisy environment.
3. Disruptive child.
4. Distracted patient.
5. Language barrier.
6. Different opinions of diagnosis, therapy, or future course.
7. Family member present who has separate agenda.
8. Patient agenda that does not match doctor's.
9. Scheduling conflict (e.g., patient schedules brief appointment and has problems requiring more time).

10. Communication equipment faulty or missing (e.g., hearing aids, teeth, glasses, etc.).
11. Patient tells saga of medical care instead of symptoms.
12. Patient has urgent needs (e.g., bedpan).
13. Patient takes interrupting phone call.
14. Differing expectation: What is the doctor's job, and what is the patient's?

Look at the case of the patient who brings a disruptive, noisy child into the interview room. Acknowledgment is simple: "I'm sorry, I am having trouble paying proper attention to your symptoms with little Charlie here kicking the furniture. Can we ask my assistant to keep him occupied out at the front desk?" This example seems very simple yet this problem is mentioned at nearly every Miles workshop and is baffling to the doctors involved.

Acknowledgment usually is accomplished by stating the problem as if it were owned by the doctor, then requesting help in resolving it. If the doctor isn't sure what needs to be done, he or she can say that, too. For example, "I'm sorry but I am having some trouble understanding just what your symptoms have been. Can you help me?" Or "I think that I am stuck here. I get the feeling that you are angry with me, yet we've never met before. Is there something going on I don't understand? Can you tell me what it is?" Or, "We seem to be tangled up somehow. I get the feeling that you are very uncomfortable with the notion that I have to examine your body. Is that true? Can you help me understand?"

Many authors have described this technique, calling it "confrontation." Physicians sometimes interpret that term as implying rude or abrupt behavior, as if they were being asked to grasp the patient's lapels and shake him. Not so. *Confrontation* has been used in the medical literature to describe the act of sharing our difficulty and requesting help. The Miles educators suggest the term *acknowledgment* as more respectful and more understandable to most of our workshop physicians.

The strategy of enlisting the patient's help in resolving interactional difficulties is a good one for many of these ex-

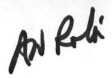

amples. For example, the patient with a list of multiple problems can be approached by a doctor who openly acknowledges
the dilemma.

Dr. X: Mr. M, I see that you have these five significant prob-
    lems. Since time is limited, I won't be able to deal with more
    than one or two today. Which would you prefer that we
    deal with now?
M: Gee, I don't know, Doc. They're all tough.
X: Yes, but I need your help. Where should we start?
M: Well, I guess I'm most concerned about the chest pain.

If this sounds too complex, we can simplify the acknowledgment process to two basic steps:

1. Agreeing on what the relationship problem is (e.g., the gum
    in his mouth)
2. Eliciting the patient's help in solving or dealing with the
    problem (e.g., spitting out the gum)

Case 15

NOTHING WRONG WITH ME

Mr. W is a 64-year-old man visiting his son 500 miles from home.
When his wife announced her intention to visit an ophthalmologist, Mr. W mentioned his failing vision. The patient's wife and
son conspired to take him along to the eye doctor, who found
a few minutes to examine him despite an already full schedule. The ophthalmologist found deep cupping, uncorrectable
vision, and increased pressure in the involved eye.

Dr. Bison: I'm afraid that I have some bad news. I think that
    you do have a problem with this eye. I think you may be
    developing glaucoma. However, since we fit you into a full
    schedule, I can't do more today. We need to do a few tests
    to confirm this diagnosis. I wonder if you would come back
    tomorrow so that we could do gonioscopy and visual fields

and recheck your pressures. I believe that it is necessary, and I always examine a patient twice before making a complete diagnosis. There will be no additional charge.

W: I don't know. I don't think I need to come back. I haven't seen a doctor for 17 years until today, and I don't believe I have to now. There's nothing wrong with me.

B: I don't understand. You came here because you were having trouble seeing.

W: Oh that's just my wife. She brought me in. There can't be anything wrong with me.

B: Well, whoever brought you, that eye isn't normal. I'll have my assistant set up an appointment for tomorrow.

W: I still don't think I need to.

Sure enough, Mr. W did not appear for his appointment the next day. But shortly, Dr. B received a request for findings from another ophthalmologist. Dr. B tried to contact Mr. W but was only able to converse with Mrs. W, who explained that he was going to see still a third doctor. Finally, months later, Dr. B found his bill returned, unpaid, with a note that said: "I'm not going to pay this. I didn't have anything wrong and I finally found a doctor who agrees with me. You caused me a great deal of stress anxiety. I had to see three more doctors, and now I have been told that I don't have glaucoma and can't get it. You charged me for the wrong diagnosis."

- What might have been done differently?
- Dr. B is still worried about his patient. He wonders about his professional responsibility at this point. Any ideas?
- The patient has called several times to discuss his bill, and the ophthalmologist agreed to "adjust it downward," but so far even that has remained unpaid. What now?

Discussion

OK, this is a good example of denial. But we meet up with denial every day. What can we do with it?

Dr. B seems to have tried to disregard the disagreement he and his patient had about the diagnosis and the need to do further tests. Since he knew that he was correct, he saw no need to do much to convince the patient at the end of their first visit. Thus they parted, disagreeing on these two vital issues. It is no surprise that the patient did not return.

I think that they needed to discuss the disagreement. If the doctor realizes that he and the patient are completely disengaged, he should make efforts to recruit his patient again. He might do something like this:

B: OK. I think I understand that we are really of two very different opinions. I think you have a real eye problem, one that we can help but that might lead to blindness if you ignore it. You think that nothing much is wrong and that it would be reasonable to do nothing more. Is that true?

W: Yeah, that's about it all right.

B: And we disagree too about what to do next. I think it would be best for you to come back tomorrow so we can recheck that eye, and you think it would be more sensible to forget all about it. Right?

W: Right again, Doc.

B: OK. What are we going to do now?

W: What do you mean?

B: I'm concerned for your welfare and for your vision. You probably are too. I can see that you are caught in a bit of a bind. You wouldn't have come here if you weren't at least a little bit concerned. But you are hesitant to go along with my ideas. What are you going to do with this dilemma?

W: Huh! I hadn't exactly thought that far. I suppose it wouldn't hurt just to come back for the tests.

B: I agree with you, Mr. Well. The tests are harmless and will give you more information to make a decision. Can I count on seeing you tomorrow?

W: OK, I guess so, Doc. When do you want me?

What happened? First the doctor articulated the diagnostic and planning disagreement that existed between doctor and patient. Then he asked the patient to engage with him to create a mutual plan, empathizing with the patient's occult dilemma. Finally he expressed his own concern for the patient. A brief conversation, but a powerful one. With such a conversation, I suspect that the patient would have returned the next day.

Dr. B might well say that he was already rushed and out of time. He had crammed this patient into a busy schedule. How could he afford the time for such a dialogue? I sympathize with his difficulty but observe that the case has taken him a lot of time and worry over the months since this event. A bit more time when the disagreement surfaced may have saved him much later.

What are the important tasks here? First, recognition that things aren't going well. This patient disagrees with his doctor on two critical elements, diagnosis and plan. Things are unlikely to get better. Second, naming the problem and putting it out between the doctor and the patient so that both can look at it. It is important to do this gently and without blame. It does no good to call the patient names or to talk about denial or noncompliance. It may be necessary to own the problem yourself and to ask the patient for help: "I'm having some difficulty here. Perhaps you can help me. I see that we are thinking two different ways and I am having a hard time finding a compromise. What do you think?"

Finally, it helps to empathize with the dilemma the patient is in: "I can see that you are caught in a bind. You are concerned about the vision in your right eye, but you really don't think much could be wrong and you are hesitant to come back to see me tomorrow. I can see that it is a tough decision for you."

I don't know what more to do about the bill. This doctor has explained to his ex-patient that the bill wasn't "for the diagnosis of glaucoma" but for the examination performed. That seems very reasonable to me. This kind doctor has even cut his fee to please this patient, a very generous offer. Maybe enough is enough. However, I am touched by the fact that the doctor and the patient seem to remain in contact by this tenuous disagreement about the bill. Maybe there will be another opportunity to discuss the more important issues, the disagreement about diagnosis and therapy, and the difficulty that Mr. Well is having coming to grips with the idea that there might be something wrong with his eye.

Case 16

A HEARING DOG

Bernice accosted the doctor at his reception desk as she saw him passing by.

B: I need to talk to you about Veronica. She needs a double prescription on all her medicines and a letter for the bus company.

Dr. Xylom: What sort of letter? What's happening?

B: She's going on a vacation. Do you remember how I told you she doesn't hear so well? The bus company will let us take our dog along if you write a letter.

X: I don't understand. Why do you need me to tell them about · the dog?

B: It's a hearing dog. It barks if someone talks to Veronica or attacks her.

Together they entered the examination room where Veronica waited. Veronica is a 45-year-old woman with a known but fairly inactive seizure disorder. She had previously been documented to have a mild hearing loss. Veronica lives with Bernice, a 60-year-old woman friend who cares for her.

X: Hello, Veronica. How are you doing?

V: Pretty good, doctor. No problems.

X: Have any seizures since I last saw you?

V: No, no seizures. But a few blackouts.

B: She blacks out.

X: How often?

V: I don't know.

B: Every so often.

V: I don't remember.

B: She had about three last month.

X: Tell me about the blackouts.

V: I don't remember them.

B: She just gets strange and sits there for a couple of minutes, and then she doesn't remember anything for about a half an hour.

X: I see. No movements or urinating or anything else?

B: No.

X: I see. Veronica, how is your hearing now?

B: She can't hear things.

V: It's OK.

X: Hmm. Well, let's retest it.

He goes out, returns with a portable audiometer, and tests her hearing, revealing the same mild hearing loss as documented six months ago.

X: Now tell me again about the dog letter.

B: We're going to Lubbock for two weeks, and the bus company won't let us take the dog unless it is a hearing or a seeing dog so you gotta write a letter.

X: Hmm. I don't know much about dogs for the hearing impaired.

B: That's OK. Just tell them we need it.

- How do you test a dog for hearing-assistance skills?
- What is the center of this doctor's distress?
- What do you think this doctor had said to his patient's caretaker on prior visits about her manipulative behavior?

Discussion

Bernice is a known manipulator. She always comes with a story that is designed to achieve some specific action by the doctor. In past years she attempted to manipulate him about issues related to her husband's care and ancillary financial support. She is fairly easy to diagnose, since she states her goal right away at the beginning of the interaction. More difficult manipulators leave their desires unstated until late in the transaction. However, in common with other manipulators, she cannot be believed. She schemes to achieve her ends as she sees them, does not trust the doctor, and cannot be trusted by the doctor.

This doctor felt himself to be at the end of his rope. He ended their relationship by telling her that he could no longer take care of her or her ward because of the manipulative behavior and because he couldn't trust her. Their final conversation went as follows:

X: Bernice, I am really troubled by all this. First of all, Veronica's hearing disorder is nowhere severe enough to qualify for a hearing-impaired dog. Second, your dog isn't trained to that task. Most important, I feel really bad about being asked to write a letter this way. I feel abused. I no longer feel I can trust what you tell me.

B: OK, if you don't want to write a letter, don't do it. I don't care.

X: No, Bernice, I think it's worse than that. I realize that I don't trust what you tell me anymore. If I don't trust you, there is no way I can be your doctor. I think you are going to have to seek medical care elsewhere. And since Veronica comes always in your charge and you provide much of her history, she'll have to find another doctor too.

B: OK, doctor. If that's what you want.

X: Yes. I'm sorry. I don't think either of you are evil people, but I just can't see how we could continue to work together.

Afterward the doctor admitted that he felt a bit guilty that he hadn't offered her a second chance, since he had never before confronted her with the issue of her manipulation. He said that he thought she probably wouldn't have been able to take advantage of a second chance but that he would have felt better about himself if he had been able to offer it. Perhaps on another day he could have done better. Perhaps he could have said something like the following:

X: Bernice, I need to talk with you about a problem I'm having. I notice that you often come to me with a very specific plan in mind and then seem to work to convince me to do that specific task. Sometimes I feel that I can't trust you to tell me the entire story because it might get in the way of your achieving your goals. Then I feel uncomfortable. I feel manipulated.

B: I'm sorry you feel that way, Doctor. I didn't mean to hurt your feelings.

X: I believe you, Bernice. But I don't think I can go on trying to be your doctor and Veronica's doctor that way. Do you think you could find a new way to work with me that is more straightforward and less manipulative?

B: What do you mean?

X: Well, what works best for me is for you to consult me about health problems and not try to get me to fix the world so that it works better for you. I especially resent it when you try to trick me into things.

B: But if I don't try to trick you, you wouldn't do it. Like the letter to the bus company about our dog.

X: That's true. On the other hand I won't do it now either. And this way I am finding it impossible to stay with you. If you want to continue with me, you will have to modify your approach.

B: I do want to keep you on for my doctor.

X: Thanks, Bernice. You see, I am beginning not to trust you. When you come here with a scheme to get me to do something I find that I lose trust in you. That makes it impossible for me to function as your doctor or Veronica's doctor. What do you think of this?

B: I don't know. I thought that patients were supposed to trust their doctors, not the other way around.

X: Yes, that's true. But it works the other way too. If either of us fails to trust the other, we can't really do anything useful for the other. So I have to be really honest with you, and you have to be more honest with me.

B: I thought I was telling you the truth. I just thought if you wrote that letter, we could take Grover along with us.

X: I see. That makes it harder for you. It sounds as if you do want to continue with me but that the issue I'm trying to describe is still puzzling to you.

B: Yeah, it is.

X: OK. Maybe we both need to think about it more. How about if I tried to tell you whenever I felt manipulated and we could take it one episode at a time?

B: OK.

What happened here? First the doctor owned the difficulty, "a problem I'm having." He described his observations and his feelings, avoiding name-calling or overt blaming. Then he asked for the patient's help—could she "find a new way to work with me?" These two steps are essential and must not be omitted for acknowledgment to be an effective process.

Case 17

KIDNEY STONE

James J, a 35-year-old attorney, became ill on Friday with minor respiratory symptoms. Only three days later did he develop left flank pain that gradually increased in severity. After three days of pain, he asked a friend for a doctor's name and appeared at Dr. Xylom's office.

X: Tell me more about the pain.

J: It has really been there for three days. It never leaves, but sometimes it does seem worse. It's there right now [pointing to left flank and into left mid-abdomen]. I can't get comfortable; I can't find any comfortable position.

X: Any other symptoms?

J: No, that's it. Just the pain. I had a stuffy head for a while but that's all gone now.

Dr. X did a careful physical examination. His patient seemed to be in pain and moved slowly. There was modest tenderness in the left flank and the left upper quadrant, but the doctor couldn't define any enlarged organs. A urinalysis showed 15 red blood cells per high power field in the spun sediment.

X: I think that you have a kidney stone. Actually the better term is a ureteral stone. A little pebble forms in the kidney and washes down into the ureter, the tube that runs from the kidney to the bladder.

J: I thought that was what it might be.

X: Right. There also may be some infection. Being partly obstructed tends to lead to infection. And sometimes the other way around. Now what I think we ought to do is take some blood tests and then send you across the street to the hospital x-ray department to do an IVP. That's an x-ray of the kidneys and all the associated plumbing. If you really have a stone, we will probably want to wait a few more days to see if it passes by itself. If not, we might have to go in there and get it out. I would want to treat you with an antibiotic and with some pain medicines. OK?

Mr. J walked across the street for his x-rays. His chest x-ray, KUB, and IVP were all quite normal. His colon and small intestine were a bit distended with gas. There were no other abnormalities. Dr. X appeared to look over the films, confer with the radiologist, and talk to his patient. He asked for an emergency kidney ultrasound and found it normal, too.

X: Hmm. Mr. J, this is very puzzling to all of us. Your story and the urinalysis led me to a diagnosis of a ureteral stone, but these x-rays don't confirm the diagnosis and don't point in any other direction. I think we ought to follow through with the plan we made across the street. Take the pain medicine and the antibiotic. Perhaps this is just a kidney infection. We'll see what the culture shows. Let's see you again in the office in two days.
J: OK, doctor.

Two days later, Mr. J felt better. The urine culture obtained on his first visit had been sterile. A repeat physical examination was normal, and a repeat urinalysis was unremarkable, now without red cells.

- What should Dr. X tell the patient about this confusion?
- How should he deal with his uncertainty regarding diagnosis and therapy?
- Should his conversation be altered in any way because this patient is a lawyer?

Discussion

Our dilemma is whether to worry the patient with our confusion or be dishonest and claim an understanding we do not have. How do patients feel when confronted with physician uncertainty? What do they say when we tell them that we don't know what's going on? How can we help them in such a bind?

The doctor can first recognize his own difficulties in an inner conversation:

X1: Oh, oh, here's trouble.
X2: What do you mean?
X1: Well first, I'm not sure what's ailing this fellow. My best efforts have led to no clear diagnosis. And he's an attorney. That's scary in itself.
X2: Yeah, I see. How do you think he feels about this?
X1: I don't know.
X2: Well, maybe you ought to find out. Remember that discovering-meaning approach?
X1: Sure. But do I want to tell him that I don't know the diagnosis?
X2: Good question! Do you?
X1: Well, it might be a good way to start. And it is the truth!
X2: OK. Go for it!

Then:

X: Well, Mr. J, by now I hope it is clear to you that we are still baffled about the diagnosis. I was pretty confident that you had a kidney stone. Now that the tests are normal, I am not sure if you had a stone that passed, an infection, or some other source of pain.

Then I think we should show understanding if the patient expresses confusion, anxiety, or anger. We can then define the usual results of such a situation and suggest further courses to follow.

X: I can imagine that no diagnosis might be worse than a nameable illness.

J: That's true, doctor. I'd almost rather have something bad and know what it is.

X: I can imagine. It might sound worrisome to have no clear diagnosis. However, I should tell you that we do find ourselves in this sort of uncertainty fairly often and that the usual result is that our patient gets well. That turns out to be better than not getting well and knowing what it was.

J: I guess so. I hope that's what happens.

X: And sometimes you don't get well so promptly but your illness declares itself in some way so that we understand it better. Right now I think we have done the appropriate studies and should just wait a little. I think that's better than subjecting you to painful or dangerous studies that are unlikely to clarify anything. We should wait a few more days, unless you become more ill. How does that sound?

This patient took his antibiotic, felt better and better, and returned to see the doctor one week later. He felt and looked well. The urinalysis was normal. Another week later he remained well. The doctor thought he'd ask his patient about the uncertainty issue.

X: Mr. J, I'm glad you have cured yourself. I wonder if you can help me understand how it felt to be in such an uncertain situation with no clear diagnosis.

J: Well, at first I was a little worried. But when the IVP was negative, I felt grateful that I wasn't going to need an operation to take out the kidney stone. Then when you did all those tests, I knew that you were being careful and thorough and weren't sloughing my problem off. And then I really appreciated your being honest with me when you didn't know what the cause of my trouble was. And I'm awfully glad that I got well again. I think you did everything just right.

Aren't we lucky that most things get better by the next morning and that most illnesses heal by themselves?

I know that many of my physician colleagues share a bias regarding attorneys, viewing them somewhat as a chicken might view a fox. But I don't think that bias should in any way color our treatment of patients, whatever their profession. We should still explain thoroughly and honor the need of patients to understand their situation and make their own decisions. In fact, I suspect that many of my colleagues treat attorneys more correctly than they do some of their other patients, and the only lesson is that they should communicate as assiduously with all their patients as they do with their lawyer-patients.

Case 18

A BOULDER KNEE

Dr. X, a Denver orthopedist, had been consulted by Mr. A about knee pain.

Mr. A: It really only hurts when I run. I do about 28 miles a week, and the last few months I had pain in my right knee much of the time. It doesn't swell up, and otherwise I'm in my usual spectacular health.

X: Well, as I said, I didn't find anything wrong on the exam, and the x-rays look fine. I think you are getting a little old for the big-time athletics you do, and that's what's bothering your knee.

A: That couldn't be, Doctor. I'm only 41. And it's only the running that hurts. I swim a mile a day and bicycle on weekends, and they don't hurt.

X: Yes . . .

A: And my chiropractor says the problem is my back alignment.

X: I remember; you told me that. But I don't see anything wrong with your back. And didn't you say that his therapy didn't help?

A: Yeah, sure. Neither did the foot massages that the reflexologist gave me or the acupuncture. Nothing's helped so far. That's why I gave up and came to you. I live in

Boulder, but I thought maybe a Denver orthopedist would be better.

X: Oh ho! I didn't know about the foot massage.

A: Well it doesn't matter; it didn't help. Nor did the Rolfing. For a while I thought the sugar-free diet was helping. My sister says I should have you look in my knee with an arthroscope.

X: Gosh. We could do that, of course, but I don't really think it would help.

A: Well, what can I do then? I don't want to cut down on the running. I'm planning to do a triathlon this summer.

X: Wow! John, my view of the knee trouble is that your knee is getting a little older, just like you are, and that your level of exercise is really more than it can take. This is an overuse syndrome.

A: How can it be overuse? I used to run 50 miles a week. Maybe I ought to go see a podiatrist. Maybe I need orthotics.

Discussion

The orthopedist thinks this patient is typical of those who come to him from Boulder, a nearby city that he thinks has more than its share of health freaks and health purveyors. I've heard similar stories from doctors in Montrose, Colorado, about patients from Telluride and from New England doctors about patients from Cape Cod. The doctors like to blame what they perceive to be a freaky atmosphere for their communication difficulty with these patients.

This doctor says half of the problem is an aging baby boomer patient, a fellow who is having trouble coming to grips with his own aging, his own frailties, and the morbidity and mortality implicit in life. Perhaps this patient is narcissistic, acting as if his deterioration is impossible or someone else's fault.

However, I think that we need to consider what we do when our diagnoses don't match our patient's, a central issue of this dialogue. This doctor thinks that his patient has a middle-aged knee that no longer can tolerate the stresses he insists on placing on it. The patient finds it unthinkable that age could be the culprit and wants a quick fix. What can they do?

The doctor could try to help his patient understand how old 41 is.

X: You know, you are not an antique. And there are surely older folk around who are still able to do amazing athletic feats. But consider: In an earlier society a 41-year-old man would be a tribal graybeard. He would no longer be a warrior. And, if your body was made to last 70 years, maybe 80 by today's standards, you are more than halfway worn out. It is OK to cut down a bit on your Olympic endeavors.

And, if that fails, the doctor could try to make his disagreement with the patient's diagnosis explicit and, acknowledging the difference, ask the patient for help in resolving their dilemma.

X: John, we are caught in a dilemma. We really have different pictures of what is going wrong and what should be done, don't we? I think your knee is wearing out a little and that at 41 you're no longer up for the Olympic endeavors you like. You think there is some specific defect that we should be able to fix to allow you to continue with your vigorous activity program.

A: Yeah, Doc, I guess we do have a difference there.

X: What can we do? How can we resolve this dilemma? Any way you see to work together?

A: I don't know, Doc. I guess that I'm really not ready to give up being young yet. I don't want to stop my athletic activities; they really are central to my life. I'm going to have to think a lot about this.

By the way, as tempting as it is, I think we have to avoid name-calling. We do ourselves and our patients damage when we lump them together and use derogatory terms like "Boulder patients" that submerge their identities and place them in a group that we view with disdain. In fact, by focusing on the dilemma of differing diagnostic opinions, this doctor does rise above the temptation to respond to a stereotype with a discount.

I admire Martin Lipp's thesis in *Respectful Treatment* [26]:

> Respect is an expression of understanding of other people, a recognition of their significance, an affirmation that what they say and do and think and experience matters to you and that you care about what happens to them and how they feel about it.

Case 19

NOSY DOCTOR

Mrs. G, a 40-year-old woman, had recently moved to town with her husband. She suffered with severe headaches that had recurred regularly for 20 years. She was told by the person who referred her that Dr. S "sometimes had success with such problems." Dr. S treated his patient with a combination of careful listening and osteopathic manipulation. He found what seemed to be a trigger spot between her scapulae and gently worked at that spot, hoping to diminish her head pain. With this care she seemed to do better and her usual headaches failed to materialize on schedule. However Dr. S thought he wasn't really getting at the cause of her trouble and began to explore her psychological and social situation. Mrs. G became very teary and refused to answer his questions.

G: Why are you asking me these questions? My previous doctors never did. I don't think they are appropriate.

S: I see. Well, it's not just because I'm a nosy doctor. I think that how you feel emotionally affects how you feel physically. Headaches often stem from an emotional conflict. It would help me to help you if I knew more about your emotional life, present and past.

G: Maybe so. But I'm not going to talk about that. I don't want to talk about those things. I just don't want to talk about those things.

She calmed down, Dr. S proceeded with his usual manipulative therapy, and she left.

On the next scheduled visit, she brought her husband, a stern, large, impressive businessman who sat in the examining room saying very little. After the manipulation therapy, the husband addressed the doctor:

Mr. G: You've made her better. No one else could do that before. I'd like to know why.

Dr. S: I can imagine that it must be puzzling to you. We think that headaches are part of a disturbed inner health state. We try to find the focus of that disturbance and use our manipulative techniques to right the disturbance. I think we've been somewhat successful with Mrs. G.

Mr. G: Yes. That seems to be helping. My wife told me that you were asking her some questions that she didn't want to answer last time. I agree. The manipulation is OK. That psychological stuff isn't. She doesn't want to talk about those things.

S: Un-huh. But you have to understand that we treat the whole patient. In fact, if we can't investigate all the potential trouble areas, I can't continue to be your wife's doctor.

Mrs. G: What? Do you mean I would have to go to another doctor? You're the only one who ever could help me.

S: Un-huh. There are two chiropractors in town who do similar manipulative therapy, and they won't ask you difficult questions. I'll be glad to give you their names.

Mr. G: We would prefer not to leave you. But if that is the only way you work, give us those names.

- What's going on? Why is this patient unwilling to discuss the matters her doctor is interested in?

- What is her husband's function in this discussion?

- Why has Dr. S decided to terminate his care of this patient? Did the decision seem a little bit sudden to you?

Discussion

Dr. S said that he suspected that Mrs. G was a childhood abuse victim and that she was having trouble "summoning up her adult" to allow her to discuss the issues now. That seems a possible hypothesis, but I have another one.

My own suspicion is that she may be a current victim of domestic violence. Her hyper-protective husband may have come in to BE SURE that critical information was suppressed. But this too is only an unfounded conjecture so far.

Dr. S said he was very surprised when this patient refused his offer of sympathetic listening. Most of his patients gladly accepted such offers. He noted that she "closed down the curtain" after her initial display of distress and then "brought in the boss," her husband, to "lay down the law." (Did Dr. S actually use all three of these clichés in one sentence? Or, was it my doing? Who knows?)

I thought that this case was surprising for at least two reasons. First, the patient was too uncomfortable to accept the offer of helpful listening at this stage, a surprise to Dr. S, but still understandable. People are ready when they are ready, not when we are. And, lacking a verbatim transcription of that interaction, I don't know if Dr. S was as helpful to his patient as he could have been. For example, after she refused to talk further about the emotional issues, he could have said:

S: I can see that it is hard for you to talk about these things. And I can hear that you think you shouldn't. But I see tears too, so I can tell you have a lot of pain that I don't yet understand. Would you be willing to help me understand this better?

And then, use of the most powerful interview tool of all, SILENCE, might have led to some fruitful disclosure.

Both Dr. S and I agree that the physician has not yet uncovered all of the patient's problem and that we need to explore further. The physician's distress with the situation in his office could have served as a tip-off to him that there was something more to discover, that something else was going on and he needed to find out what it was.

Childhood sexual abuse and domestic violence leave their victims with issues of trust and control. So many of our female patients are likely to have been violated in some way that physicians must include questions about abuse in order to have complete physical data. The patient may take some time, however, to feel enough trust in her physician to discuss her situation.

An important difference between the victim of childhood abuse and the battered spouse lies in the spouse's current danger. She may be in a potentially lethal situation and may feel trapped. She may be afraid to disclose anything for fear of retribution by her spouse.

All this is of course still conjectural. We need more data, and Dr. S seems to have cut off the possibility that it will be he who will turn up the needed information. Why did that happen? And what is the reason for Dr. S's inflexibility? This usually flexible physician became adamant when the patient and her husband refused to play by his rules. It was "my rules or I take my bat and ball and go home." What accounted for his inflexibility? What usually accounts for our inflexibilities? I can imagine several possibilities:

1. The doctor is always inflexible. Some pseudo-physicians, usually more technician than doctor, can never bend very much.

2. Perhaps the doctor was already angry with this patient or overextended. This last event may be the last straw.

3. There are no other options for treatment. (Pretty unlikely!)

4. This may be an idiosyncratic area for this particular doctor. For him, perhaps this is the only route he can see for such a patient. We all have areas that we cannot deal with.

5. The doctor may have painted himself into a corner. I think this is the most common explanation for our inflexibilities. We are having a bad day, pop out a single plan, and seem stuck to it. When we do this and later realize what we have done, we need to apologize. The apology may be late; it usually takes me several days to realize what I have done, but late is better than never.

Once we discussed this differential diagnosis for doctor rigidity, Dr. S decided that his experience was a variant of the last category. He said that he was more annoyed than he realized at the time, not by the patient's unwillingness to play by his rules, but by the husband's presence and threatening posture. He thought they demonstrated a lack of trust, something that always pains him. And the feeling he had of becoming a victim to the powerful husband angered him. So he threw the patient out of his practice, perhaps a symbol for what he would have liked to do to the husband—toss him out of the office.

Well, what now? What will Dr. S do about this interaction? He might choose to do nothing, letting not-well-enough alone. Or he might just file away in his memory the fact that he acted less rationally than he'd like when threatened by a bully. Or he might call up the couple for another interview. He could choose to reaccept the patient on her terms, leaving the invitation for further emotional exploration open for the future should she decide to trust him with her feelings. Or he could actually discuss his own feelings with the couple, explaining what the doctor feels when his patients trust him less than he thinks they should. As you might guess, I like this fourth option best. But maybe it's not best for Dr. S. All I am sure of is that the physician cannot even see these potential avenues until he addresses the question of "Why did I suddenly become so uncharacteristically inflexible?"

Case 20

NOT CHEMICALS

Mr. A usually consults Dr. Y. Because Dr. Y is on vacation, his partner, Dr. X, was seeing Mr. A for the first time. Trying to be two doctors at once led Dr. X to feel rushed and out of sorts. The doctor's office assistant had already assiduously compiled a list of current therapies.

X: Mr. A, I see that you are taking a whole lot of medications.
A: No, doctor, I only take the AZT and the acyclovir and the ketoconazole. The others are Shackley products; they're all natural.
X: I see listed Halcion, vitamin E, beta-carotene, zinc, Herblax, Formula One, EPA, vitamin C, lecithin, vitamin B, calcium,

magnesium, aloe vera juice, Bumex, Dyazide, aspirin, and Empirin.

A: Oh, yeah, I forgot the Halcion and the diuretics.

X: And the others? What is EPA by the way?

A: That's just fish emulsion. It's natural.

X: Anything else?

A: Well I did want to ask you about this Duofilm that I've been using on my foot.

X: OK. Well I have to tell you that I have no idea what is in several of these and no idea if they are interfering with anything else you are taking.

A: They couldn't, doctor; they aren't chemicals.

X: Not chemicals?

A: That's right.

X: That's ridiculous. Everything is chemicals, including you and me.

A: No, I've studied this, and I know they are not. I discussed it all with an endocrinologist, and she agreed with me.

X: OK, and the problem you came in for today was?

A: I guess first of all it was the neuropathy. I've been having weakness in my legs, and my right knee gives way. So I stopped the DDI about a week ago. I wonder if DDC is available yet. My T_4 cell count had been in the 200s and now is 363 so I think the DDI was helping, but I was worried about the neuropathy and that last lab test when my CPK was over a thousand.

X: So you're worried about the blood tests and about your leg weakness.

A: Yes, and I wonder if you ought to increase the AZT dosage or start DDC. I've been drinking a lot of Mylanta for my stomach.

X: Mylanta? Are there any other drugs you're taking that we haven't listed yet?

A: No, that's it. And, doctor, I told you most of these aren't drugs.

X: [Irate] OK, I understand that's how you look at them, but I have to tell you that they are all drugs and they are either placebos or they have potential side effects, and no one, not me or Dr. Y or anyone else, can sort out a muddle like this. In the meantime, I better look at your legs and your stomach. I need you to climb out of your clothes and sit up on this examining table. You can keep your shorts on and cover up with this sheet. I'll be back in a minute or two.

• What do you think is Dr. X's first task at this time?

Discussion

Sure, patients have little sense of the chemical nature of everything they put into their bodies. And sure, we aren't very good at sorting out combination effects of drugs that we understand well, much less those of whose contents we are ignorant.

But the big problem is that Dr. X is losing his patience and becoming angry and intolerant of his patient's health theories. It's one thing to explain your needs and your abilities and quite another to become angry with the patient for transgressing your limits.

I think the task for this doctor is apology. Then he has to try a new skill—patience and containment of his strong feelings.

X: I'm back, Mr. A. But before I examine you I want to apologize and ask your forgiveness. I have been cross and irritable, and that is inappropriate. I'm sorry. I will try to do better.

A: That's OK, doctor. I told you they weren't chemicals.

X: Hmm. Well, I want you to understand that I apologize for my bad manners. But I do have to say that I still view all the remedies as possible hazards and possibly dangerous as they mix together in the body. Now maybe we ought go on to the examination.

A: OK, doctor.

Our work is difficult and often very frustrating. It is not surprising that we occasionally lose our tempers. But such a loss is antitherapeutic, and we must do what we can to recoup. There is nothing as good as an apology in such a situation. Then we have to try to pull ourselves together and do better.

This doctor couldn't quite manage a pure apology but felt obliged to incorporate it with a further restatement of his intellectual position. Well, better than nothing, I guess. On a really good day, he could probably have stopped with the apology. Of course, on a really good day he might not have dug himself into such a hole to start with.

Case 21

I SHOULDN'T HAVE BEEN CHARGED SO MUCH

Susan brought her husband in to Dr. X for his routine postoperative visit. She and her husband were feeling fine. They both asked for "flu shots," and the doctor authorized them even though he was not Susan's doctor.

One week later, Susan called for an emergency appointment. She had been sick since the influenza vaccination with aches, mild fevers, and malaise. She needed "only a few minutes," she said, since it was just a "touch of the flu." When she did appear in the office she gave no other significant history except that her grandson had been ill with cough, fever, and aches about four days before her influenza vaccination and that she had spent a day in the grandson's company when he was sick. The doctor examined her carefully; the physical examination was completely normal. She appeared to be less lively than usual, but there were no other abnormal findings. She was given a diagnosis of a "viral flu-like syndrome" and sent home with recommendations for acetaminophen and rest. Dr. X drew a CBC out of curiosity and explained that the influenza vaccine was not a live virus and couldn't give her "the flu." He thought that she had caught her illness from her grandson.

The next day she called the office quite irate. She had read her bill and discovered that it listed her visit as a "new patient, complete examination" and charged $110. She said that she shouldn't have been charged so much. "I wasn't that sick!" she said. The receptionist explained that the charges weren't proportionate to the patient's illness severity but to the amount of time the doctor spent. "Nonetheless," Susan said, "I wasn't sick enough. He should have charged less."

The following day, a Saturday, she called Dr. X and said that she was worse, having developed bilateral pleuritic chest pain. He recommended that she try ibuprofen and promised to call her on Sunday. Indeed, the next day, he called her to learn that the pain was much better. On Monday morning, the doctor found her chart on his desk, with the receptionist's note about her call on Friday, complaining about the bill. He also found the laboratory test returned. She had a white cell count of 18,000 with 80% mature neutrophils and 15% band forms. The doctor called her again. She reported that the chest pain was manageable but that it was still present. She agreed to come to the office on Tuesday.

On Tuesday morning she arrived, feeling "pretty bad all over." The doctor could now hear bilateral loud rales both anterior and posterior in her lungs. However she was afebrile, she had no sputum, and her oxygen saturation was 95%. The two discussed the possibility of a viral pneumonia and how they might continue to treat it at home if she wished. Then the doctor sent her across the street to a radiology facility for a chest x-ray. At his lunchtime he walked over to look at the films and confer with a radiologist. The x-ray showed fluffy reticular infiltrates in both lungs. Dr. X found his patient waiting in the radiology suite.

X: Well Susan, you do have what looks like a pneumonia. Come look at these films.

They examined the x-ray films together, the doctor pointing out the infiltrates. Then they again discussed their plans for the next few days.

X: Oh, by the way, Susan, I noted that you called to complain about the bill.
S: Oh, doctor, please disregard that call. You have spent so much time with me the last four days, and all those phone calls. I'm sorry I complained.
X: That's all right, Susan. But you know how you said that you weren't sick enough for such a big charge?

S: Oh, doctor, I'm sorry I ever said that. I hope you forget all about it.

X: Well, what I think we know now is that you are a lot sicker than we thought you were. I better go back to the office and double the bill!

- Should our medical charges parallel the patient's disease severity?

- Should we charge for our services only if we get the patient well?

- Should our charges be small when we just spend time with the patient? When we think more than we act? When we don't do procedures?

- How can this doctor keep his mind on his doctoring and less on his banking?

Discussion

This outrageous comment by a physician who has just begun to care for his new patient may seem too much to tolerate. Fortunately Dr. X already had a good relationship with Susan because of their long contacts during her husband's illness the preceding year. And sometimes outrageous comments can be therapeutic. If the doctor can see something to chuckle about, perhaps the situation isn't altogether hopeless.

Is this case really about our confused system of financing medical care? This internist feels discounted and unfairly treated when he considers that his thoughtful, careful time is recompensed at an hourly rate about one-twentieth of that of his ophthalmologist or orthopedist colleagues. He is likely to come unglued when medical economics are the focus of his attention.

I believe that we need to acknowledge these sources of concern to ourselves. If we become focused on financial issues, we may lose sight of everything else. But we can't avoid such a focus unless we acknowledge to ourselves our own concern.

Earle P. Scarlett's essay "What Is a Profession?" says it well [27]:

> We in the medical profession are at times apt to be confused and have our attention distracted by the temper and spectacle of the contemporary scene. There is plenty of talk about medical economics, but less about the philosophical aspects of our craft. To be sure, we cannot be indifferent to changing economic conditions or to the technical needs of the community which we serve. But we must look to our own household and keep it in order.

Scarlett defined "seven pillars" of our profession: technical skill and craftmanship, a sense of social responsibility with an interest in community life, a knowledge of history, a knowledge of literature and the arts, personal integrity, a faith in meaning and value of life, and the grace of humility. He said that these made for the equilibrium of mind that is the mark of the professional person. Their expression in action and thought were what Scarlett thought made the profession great.

Our take-home income is nowhere in this list. Somehow we have to try to put our financial issues in perspective! And how necessary it is to do so to remain a physician!

Case 22

DIALYSIS

The patient was 35 years old and suffered from a rapidly progressive chronic renal failure. He had hematuria, anemia, and required considerable medical attention as well as chronic dialysis. However, he was uncooperative, seldom followed instructions, and was abusive to staff and physicians alike. He was particularly difficult for the dialysis unit director, a female physician.

Dr. A: How are you today, Mr. S?

S: Bug off.

A: You know that I have to be here to supervise your dialysis, don't you?

S: Yeah. Do me a favor. Supervise from farther away. I've had it with you and the rest of the broads here.

Dr. A says that she has tried logic, joking, anger, and finally semi-abandonment. She now has given up and tries to avoid this patient, leaving his usual care to his primary care physician, who seems to manage by mirroring Mr. S's moods and comments. If Mr. S is abusive, Dr. K abuses him back. Yet Dr. A thinks that Mr. S is not receiving as good care as he would if she were more involved. She has asked several colleagues for their ideas. They have suggested that she has done well by backing out. One colleague suggests telling Mr. S to "shape up or ship out."

- What do you think?

Discussion

This case reminds me of a CPC in the *New England Journal of Medicine* several years ago. The patient then was also a young man who did not cooperate with his doctors, signed out of the hospital against medical advice, and eventually died of his renal disease. I recall writing a letter to the editor suggesting that the discussion of the case, dealing only with his renal disease, might have been expanded to deal with the intransigence and uncooperativeness of the patient, features that killed him as much as did his kidney disease. The letter was not published. I took it to be a statement of the times. I believe that doctors and editors are now more aware that doctor-patient communication phenomena influence our medical results.

But what more could Dr. A do? She seems to have tried everything. However, she might try one more confrontation with the patient.

A: Mr. S, I wonder if you have noticed that I haven't been visiting with you on your last few dialysis treatments.
S: Yeah. Good riddance, I say.
A: Well, I thought that you might like to understand why I have been more distant and that you might like to consider the matter again.
S: Yeah?

A: I have found it hard to deal with your abusive behavior, so I have withdrawn. I am content to give technical direction from a distance. Of course, that is not as good for you than if I took a more active interest in your case.

S: What's wrong with Dr. Kindly? He's my doctor.

A: That's true, and Dr. Kindly is a fine man and an excellent physician. I'm more trained in working with kidney diseases though.

S: So I don't do so well if you aren't caring for me?

A: True.

S: What's the big deal? How come you're ignoring me? Doctors aren't supposed to abandon their patients.

A: I told you. I can't cope with abusive behavior. If I am to continue with you, we have to have some ground rules on how we treat each other.

S: Shit!

A: Fine. I just wanted to explain my position.

S: Wait a minute; don't go off. Maybe I can do what you want. Just what is it that bothers you?

Is this far-fetched? Maybe so. But it might work, and I think Dr. A could try it. Dr. A has nothing to lose by giving this a try. She might even ask the patient if he feels she has done anything to upset him at any point. Who knows?

What else? She might recruit Dr. Kindly to explain her position with the patient. And, indeed, her present position of technical supervision from a distance isn't so bad, even though it will require more communication between herself and Dr. Kindly.

Case 23

MY NECK HURTS

Dr. C: Hello Ms. Robin, what brings you to me?

R: I have this terrible pain in my neck, doctor.

C: Uh, huh?

R: And it interferes with my work. I have to stay home some days.

C: I see. But I'm a plastic surgeon. Why are you consulting me about this trouble?

R: Well, I'm sure that the pain is because of my breasts. They're too large and heavy, and Dr. Smith said maybe they're causing my neck pain. He says you do excellent work at breast reduction, and that's what I want.

C: I see. Well, yes, I do that, and I would be glad to help you. Of course, I'm not sure that the breasts are the cause of your neck pain; I couldn't guarantee that reduction surgery would help your pain.

R: Oh, you wouldn't have to do that Doctor. Just be sure to tell the insurance company that you're doing the operation for neck pain. Then they will pay for it.

C: You want me to tell your insurance company that we are operating to help your neck trouble . . .

R: Yes, Doctor. Otherwise they call it cosmetic surgery and won't pay. That's what I learned when I talked with Dr. Form in Denver. He's another breast surgeon. He said it was cosmetic surgery and I would have to pay myself. But Dr. Smith says that the insurance will pay as long as I have a diagnosis.

C: I see.

- What do you think? Will the breast reduction help Ms. R's neck pain?

- Are you willing to tell a little white lie to support Ms. R's needs? After all, the breast reduction will surely make her happier, and perhaps if she is better off psychologically, the neck pain will go away.

- In general, what do doctors do when asked to fudge on the facts to help their patients?

Discussion

Dr. C says that this sort of request is one of the most difficult problems he faces in his practice of plastic and reconstructive surgery. He knows that a lot of his work is cosmetic, and he is proud of the work he does. But he doesn't like having to lie to anyone, including the insurance company. And he feels that he is being manipulated by a patient who asks him to do this. Yet he knows that there may even be a psychological, if not physical, connection between her concern that her breasts are too large and her neck pain.

We all know that we are liable for all sorts of punishment if we falsify records or perjure ourselves. And we have strong moral training against such falsehoods. But many physicians also feel that their primary loyalty is to their patients and are less concerned about insurance company rules. They may believe, along with Ivan Illich [28], that the most dangerous doctor is the "incorruptible professional" who cannot bend any rule no matter how important it is to his patient. Illich would argue for situational ethics, a need to decide each case on its merits no matter how strong the overarching principles. I do suspect that Illich would have less sympathy with a patient desiring cosmetic surgery than with many other possible instances, but even here, he might say one must consider the individual situation.

I wonder too if sometimes we are more inclined to bend toward the patient's wishes to deceive the insurance company if our own economy is suffering. Would the surgeon be more willing to tell this "little white lie" if he "needed the business"?

Novack et al. [29] recently studied how physicians would behave when lying seemed to produce a better patient outcome. They found most physicians willing to bend the truth to get a mammogram for a patient, but even more willing to lie to defend themselves from threats of malpractice.

Whatever you or I would do, Dr. C is clear that he does not want to falsify his view of the matter to the insurance company. What he wants is a way to discuss the matter with his patient. I think he has to speak from the "I" position, avoid name-calling, and be forthright.

C: Ms. R, I'm afraid that I can't do exactly what you are asking. I feel comfortable doing the surgery if you wish, but because I am so unsure of the connection between the size of your breasts and your neck pain, I couldn't tell the insurance company that was the reason.

R: But then they won't pay.

C: Yes, that's true.

R. But Dr. Smith says the breasts are causing my pain.

C: I know. But I am much less sure than he was. I can imagine that it is very aggravating for you to hear this.

R: I can't afford the breast surgery myself.

C: I see.

R: And I am so tired of being this way. I've never liked the way I look this way.

C: I can understand your distress.

Of course there is also the possibility that Dr. C might want to do some negotiation about the price. Maybe that's really the prime issue.

Case 24

OLIVE OIL

Dr. W: Hello, Mrs. Pain. How have you been doing?

P: Not too hot, Doctor. I still have those episodes when my gallbladder acts up.

W: Same old thing?

P: Yes. Only they are getting more often now. I get pain spells a couple of times a week. Last week I woke up with that side pain and had to walk around for an hour or so three nights in a row. Last night was the first time I slept through. I'm really tired in the morning when that happens. I wonder if you can give me some sort of a tonic so I'll have more energy in the daytime.

W: A tonic? You need to have your gallbladder removed. Then those stones won't wake you up and you'll have enough energy.

P: Oh Doctor, you know I don't want to have surgery. I'm going to dissolve the stones. I've switched to pure olive oil, and my nutritionist says that will probably just dissolve those old stones right away.

W: Your nutritionist doesn't know what she's talking about. That's a bunch of hooey.

P: He! My nutritionist is a man, Doctor. And he's certified.

W: He might be a certified looney for all I care. You need an operation.

P: That isn't true, Doctor. I read in *Prevention* magazine that gallstones can be dissolved away and that doctors just make a lot of money taking out gallbladders.

W: Look, you can sometimes dissolve stones with medication, but it's dangerous for someone like you who has a lot of middle-sized stones. They might just get small enough to lodge in your common bile duct. And olive oil isn't the way.

P: It's extra virgin olive oil.

W: I don't care what its morals are. Olives won't do it. I'll bet you ten to one.

P: I don't bet, Doctor. I don't smoke or drink or bet. And I'm surprised at you for suggesting such a thing.

W: OK, I give up. What can I do for you today?

P: Nothing, Doctor, I just wanted to come by and say hello. Except maybe you can give me another prescription for the pain medicines. They help a little.

• Do you ever get into an argument with your patients about diagnoses or therapy?

• Do you bet on the outcome? If so, do you bet with or against your patient?

• Any suggestions for Dr. W?

Discussion

We do disagree with our patients, usually about the facts of the case (often because we didn't check back with the patient to see that the story we heard was the story she told), the diagnoses, and the therapy. When we have such a disagreement, arguing seldom helps. What we need to do is to identify the points of conflict and let the patient know that we know we are stuck.

W: Well, Ms. P, I think we are stuck here.

P: What do you mean, Doctor?

W: We don't agree on what is the best thing to do. I think your gallstones are dangerous to you, might go on to cause something awful like inflammation of your pancreas or gallbladder, what we call acute pancreatitis or acute cholecystitis, and need to be fixed soon. And I think that surgery is the only way to go. You think that you can dissolve the stones with olive oil.

P: That's what my nutritionist says, too.

W: So we have a real disagreement. What are we going to do?

P: I don't understand.

W: Well, I am really concerned with your welfare, and I do have some technical knowledge that comes from many years of medical training. I am afraid that you are being misled and will be in more danger if you put the surgery off.

P: You don't think the olive oil will help.

W: I really don't.

P: Well, I'll still have to think about it some more.

W: I wish you would. You know, Ms. P, I have cared for you for a long time, and I really hate to think of you having something bad happen when we could head it off in time if we just acted sooner.

P: I appreciate that, Doctor. It's just that I'm scared of surgery.

W: Yes. You know, I don't think I really considered that fully before. Can you tell me more about just what frightens you?

Aha! Now we're getting somewhere. Maybe it's what Dr. W doesn't know that is the key. Maybe the conflict about the olive oil isn't as important as understanding what his patient's fears are.

I think there is another important issue to address—Dr. W's anger. I can imagine how he would be angry with a patient who gave more credence to a pseudo-expert than to him, but his anger blocks his ability to explore her point of view. He needs to stop, identify his own feelings, control his defensiveness, and then focus on his patient's issues.

It might be necessary for Dr. W to have a silent discussion with himself before he says anything to this patient:

W1: Hold on a second, W. You sound pretty angry.

W2: I'm not angry. This woman is just full of hooey.

W1: Wait a minute. Listen to yourself talk: terms like "hooey," "looney," "I don't care what its morals are."

W2: Well, I guess that I am a little steamed. She does that to me.

W1: OK. Any idea what it is that she does that is so tough for you?

W2: Well, first she doesn't give me any credit for knowing anything and listens to any quack she can find.

W1: So she discounts your expertise.

W2: Yeah. Like all my medical training is worth nothing.

W1: You feel a lot discounted by her.

W2: That's right. And I am worried about her.

W1: Worried?

W2: Yeah. One of these nights she's going to get really sick with cholecystitis, and I'll have to get up in the middle of the night to operate on her.

W1: She'll become an even bigger nuisance.

W2: Yeah. And the surgery will probably be difficult; maybe she'll have some complication, and she'll probably blame me.

W1: You've got quite a scenario figured out.

W2: I guess I do.

W1: Anything else?

W2: No. I think that's it. I guess I am mad at her.

Once that internal dialogue is finished, Dr. W may be ready to talk with his patient. He might want to tell his patient some of this or he might not. If he thought her capable of being empathic and he trusted her, he might let her in on his secret.

W: I think I understand what's troubling me, Ms. P.

P: You want me to have an operation?

W: Yes, that's true. But what I meant was that I found that I was getting unsettled as you were telling me what you've been doing. I think I was getting angry. And I don't think you're to blame for my feelings.

P: I wondered if you were mad at me.

W: I can imagine. And I apologize if I let some of that feeling slip out. I think that I have a hard time sometimes when it seems to me as if my patient is valuing my diligent care and hard-acquired knowledge very little and is taking advice from a caregiver who is much less well trained.

P: Like the nutritionist?

W: Yes. But you know, that's my issue, not yours. I don't have to burden you with it.

P: I guess we're all human, Dr. W. It's nice of you to tell me.

I believe that this doctor then needs to understand why his patient is unwilling to follow his advice. There is something left to find out. *More understanding is needed, not more persuasion.* How common that is! We try to persuade when we still don't understand. We need to discover the meaning of all this. "Can you tell me more about what frightens you?" might lead to the heart of the matter. We can ask all sorts of meaning questions like "What do you think might happen if we did an operation?", "With whom else have you talked about surgery?", "Has anyone else you know had to go through surgery like this?", "How has this trouble with your gallbladder affected your life so far?", "Is this illness affecting your life? Your hopes for the future? Your work? Your family? How so?"

I don't know exactly where this discussion would go with Ms. P. But I am sure that until we discover what this illness and this recommended therapy mean to her, we won't get past the roadblock. Time to find out.

So what am I talking about? Acknowledging a difficulty? Or discovering meaning? BOTH of course! No one technique completely excludes another.

4

So What Else Is New?

I'm on my way out, my hand on the doorknob, and she says to me, "By the way, Doctor. . . ."

Dr. Xylom

Common things are common.

Old doctors' saying

Everybody's doing it, doing it, doing it.
Irving Berlin, "Everybody's Doing It Now," 1912

What was everybody doing in 1912? The Turkey Trot, of course.

Several common patient communication syndromes seem to annoy doctors more than they would if the doctors just realized that they were so common. Consider this list:

1. The patient who comes with his own diagnosis (often known as a "theorist").
2. The patient who brings his own idea of correct therapy.
3. The patient who presents with multiple complaints, a list of complaints, or who, at the last minute, reveals his most serious ailment, which he has not mentioned until that moment (the "doorknob syndrome" or the "by-the-way patient").
4. The patient who tells his theory of causation instead of

answering the doctor's questions about timing and location of symptoms.

5. The patient who has an extensive list of questions that he needs answered before you can get him out of the office.

6. The patient who has consulted with three relatives, a pharmacist, a chiropractor, and a neighbor who is a nurse before coming to see you.

7. The patient who is following your recommendations but also seeking help from an acupuncturist and a herbalist.

8. The patient who talks about the "illness" rather than his "disease." The illness is presented in a narrative that includes theories of etiology and descriptions of consequences. People are mentioned who seem, to the physician, not to fit into the narrative.

9. The patient who does not follow the doctor's advice because he hasn't yet been enlisted in that sort of action, presenting as a "noncompliant patient," "passive patient," "unresponsible for lifestyle," and "unwilling to change his behavior."

The common theme is that these are all so very common. All of us have our own explanatory models or diagnoses in mind before we come to see the doctor. All of us have at least an idea of what correct therapy might be. Most have consulted several other people including family members and nonphysicians. There are more annual visits to "nonstandard" health care givers than there are to primary care doctors [30]. Lots of our patients are also consulting a naturopath, an acupuncturist, an herb doctor, and a chiropractor. Most of our patients have multiple complaints, probably averaging about three.

Sometimes we begin to think of ourselves as victims and the patient as the agent of our torture. It is sometimes hard to accept that patients are never there to meet our needs for clarity, precision, and cooperation. They are focused only on their own needs, and rightfully so. Serving others all day, day after day, as we do, isn't easy. It helps to develop some ways of nurturing ourselves while we respond to others. I like to collect examples of patients' behavior, so when a patient tells me that his problem is "too much poison in his system," I add another gem to my collection of explanatory models and write in the chart, "E.M. = too much poison in the system." Much more enjoyable than being pained with every patient who comes bearing an E.M.—a number that turns out to be 100%, if I only look.

The dialogue that follows will show you what I mean.

Case 25

IT ALL BEGAN IN 1949

Dr. X: Hi! I'm Dr. Xylom. I understand that you were referred by Patty First.

R: Yes, doctor. I'm Robert Ruth. Patty said she thought I ought to come see you.

X: Uh huh. What sort of trouble have you been having?

R: Well, doctor, it all began in 1949. I was up camping in the San Juans. We had been elk hunting, but my Uncle Phil couldn't come with us that year because he was having tax troubles.

X: Wait, Mr. Ruth, I think maybe we ought to start at the other end. This is 1994. Maybe you could start with what's happening now.

R: Well, I would, but to understand it, you have to start at the beginning. See, Phil, he used to take care of all our stuff. He'd arrange the tents and the sleeping bags and all. Then when he got busy and then he got sent to prison, we went without him and we didn't get things arranged as well.

X: And now you . . .

R: Well, we didn't have the right sleeping bags, and we all caught colds. I was only 11 then, but I was pretty sick, I guess. When I got home, I was so sick that my mother took me to the doctor, and he gave me a big shot of penicillin. Even then I was home from school for a week or so.

X: OK, I see. But perhaps if you could tell me how you are now and then we could . . .

R: Well, ever since that time, I've been easy to catch colds or bronchitis. So, anyway, I've had this bronchial condition that comes on and . . .

X: Is it causing trouble right now?

R: I'm getting there, Doctor. Hold your horses.

X: Oh.

R: Well, I keep having this cough that comes on every spring, and I've had to come for antibiotics most years. Dr. Calm said that I would probably continue to have this unless I stopped smoking, but I figure it was that trip to the mountains that did me in. If I hadn't used the wrong sleeping bag and got wet, I probably wouldn't be in the fix I'm in now.

X: You are still smoking?

R: Yeah, but not that much.

X: And what sort of trouble are you having now?

R: It's the same thing, doctor. I keep coughing. Sometimes I think I'm going to cough my lungs up.

Case 26

I'M SICK, DOCTOR

Estelle has come to see her doctor on her regular every-two-week visit. She is 70 years old and has been consulting Dr. Ready for ten years. Her doctor has never been able to understand just how she is feeling unwell. Physical examination and laboratory testing have revealed no abnormalities. She has changed not a whit during the last ten years. This visit is no different from her usual.

Dr. R: Hello, Estelle, how are you doing?

E: I'm sick, doctor. I'm sick.

R: Uh-huh. And can you tell me what sort of symptoms you are having?

E: It's just like always, doctor. I just don't feel well. I'm sick.

R: I see. Is this mostly a matter of pain? Of nausea? Of fatigue? What is it mostly?

E: Not really any of those, doctor. I'm just so very sick.

R: Has it interfered with anything you do?

E: I can't do anything, doctor. I'm too sick. I stay home during the day, while my son John works. His wife, Cathy, works too. They come home at night. I'm sick.

R: I see. Have you been eating all right?

E: About the same as usual, doctor. I don't eat much. I'm just too sick.

R: What about your bowels?

E: They're terrible, just like always. I never have a bowel movement. I'm too sick.

The interview proceeded in this fashion for a few more minutes. Then Dr. R suggested that he do an examination. A partial physical examination was, as in the past, unrevealing.

R: Well, I don't find anything wrong. I think you should just keep doing what you are doing. I will see you in a while.

E: When should I come back, doctor? I don't think it should be more than a few weeks. I'm not well, you know.

- What's wrong with this patient?
- What does this doctor want to do for her?
- What can he do?

Discussion

This doctor says he felt frustrated with this patient for ten years. Finally he retired and willed her to his successor. He was always bothered by his inability to get any specific symptomatology from her, to find anything to treat, and to be able to fix anything. To make matters worse, he could never keep her from reappearing at his office within a few weeks with exactly the same refrain.

So what is going on?

One feature of this case is its veterinary aspect, a common phenomenon when the history is unavailable or useless. (In this category are patients who are unable to give us historical data, who give too much positive data, or who have "positive review of systems histories" and patients who are confused, demented, or unconscious.) This problem is hardest to comprehend when the patient seems alert and coherent but unable to find or describe symptoms.

One must wonder what "I'm sick, doctor" really means. We usually think first of the disease model. It might be better to use a disability model or a personality model with this patient. The English language limits us by providing only one verb *to be*. In many languages, subtleties can be clarified by two verbs. Spanish uses *ser* to mean a permanent state and *estar* to mean one that is more transient. If a person claimed, "Estoy enfermo" ("I am sick"), we would assume he meant a temporary illness. If he said, "Soy enfermo," we would translate it to mean "I am sickly," a permanent state. I think that the patient in this vignette is really describing a permanent state. She is "sickly" and thus unable to cope with the exigencies of life. She no more expects the doctor to repair that deficit than to fly to the moon.

What can the doctor do? He can recognize the patient's picture of her state.

R: I see that you still are quite sick, Estelle. I don't find anything new wrong, and I don't think you are in any worse shape, but I suspect that you are in the same condition as before. I doubt that we can do anything to make it better. You will have to continue bearing up even though you feel so bad.

E: I know, doctor. I don't ever expect to get better. I'm just too sick for that.

The most therapeutic response we can make here is to applaud her bearing up. Considering her perception of her health, she is doing the best she can.

And why does she keep coming back?

Perhaps she has some underlying anxiety that feeling as bad as she does, as incapable of any activity, some awful disease is lurking. If so, the doctor's regular examinations and reassurances may keep her anxiety at a tolerable level. She may also need regular reassurance that the doctor understands how bad she feels and how unable she is to function.

Is this really a case of occult chronic depression? Maybe. But if so it is a very long-lasting depression and probably will not respond to any therapy. I would be tempted to try treating her with an antidepressant medication, but I wouldn't expect miracles. Perhaps Prozac might help, as it often does in subtle characterologic disorders, but I haven't found it very helpful in my older patients who are "always sick."

There may be a number of depression equivalents that we see in our offices. My neurologist friends tell me that one of the most common complaints they see is dizziness. They say that the true diagnosis is often depression. And the chronic fatigue that presents so often to an internist may also stem from depression. Unfortunately, in my experience such symptoms only occasionally respond to antidepressant medication and even less often to psychotherapy. In the end we are often left with this "familiar face syndrome" and find that the best we can do is affirm the patient's distress and her efforts to function as well as she can, then not meddle too much. Dr. Tim Hopf says that his principle in such cases is "Don't just do something; stand there." That sounds right to me.

Case 27

NO STARCH

Dr. M: Mr. B, what brought you into the hospital?

B: I had swollen legs. My wife insisted I come here.

M: How did it happen?

B: The swelling began about a year ago. I had been working as a security supervisor and my legs just started swelling.

M: Any other problems?

B: Nope. Just that my wife said I had to come in and get the swelling looked at. She took me to Dr. K, and he said it was too much for him, so he sent me to the cardiologist, Dr. Q.

M: From your point of view, then, you didn't feel that bad?

B: Well yeah, dizzy sometimes. I'd get light-headed.

M: Any other problems? Chest pain or shortness of breath?

B: Just when I go up stairs. I get winded, and I have to lean on the banister.

M: Any other problems? Pain? Pressure?

B: No. I always have lung trouble though. I use 3S Tonic to thin the blood.

M: Thin your blood?

B: Yeah. I have this plasma problem. It thickens up. So I have a starch-free diet. I have to avoid starch. No starch.

M: Anything else?

B: Just my gallbladder. They took that out twice. And a hernia once. I was OK until I passed out on the creeper. I woke up in the hospital, and they had taken out my gallbladder.

M: That must have been quite a shock.

- What's going on?
- What is this patient's view of his medical problems?
- What's a creeper?

Discussion

Sometimes our patients tell such chaotic stories that we have trouble following them. When we are lost in space, it often helps to ask the patient to focus on symptoms. Then we can seek clarification from the real eyewitness, the patient who experiences the symptoms. But I have to admit that a lot of the color and fun in my work comes from my patients' ideas of pathophysiology. Mr. B has some wonderful ideas, my favorite being his idea that starch would thicken up his blood. I guess that makes sense; it stiffens up his shirt collars.

I also have the feeling that this patient views his medical issues as a huge mystery. Things happen to him that he really does not understand. He has had to come to the hospital because of a serious problem of which he was more or less unconscious. And once, on his "creeper," a platform on wheels that he uses to roll about under the cars he is repairing, he did pass out and ended up in the hospital. I would be tempted to tell him that it sounds to me as if medical matters often come as big surprises to him. He'd probably be glad to know that we understood how it seemed to him. Then we could explore for reasons: Is he confused? Is he denying the significance of symptoms that he is aware of? We'll have to get him focused on symptoms to find out.

How might this go? Something like this:

M: Mr. B, as you describe these medical events, I sense that several have come as really big surprises to you. It sounds as if they just came bang out of the blue.

B: You aren't kidding, Doc. One minute I'm well, and the next I'm hooked up to the cardiogram and the intravenous.

M: Wow! That does sound surprising. One other thing that has me confused is this—were there no symptoms at all besides the dizziness and leg swelling?

B: What do you mean, "symptoms," Doc?

M: Well, pain or shortness of breath or itch or nausea or . . .

B: Oh sure. I was pretty winded, like I said. That and dizzy.

M: OK, I see. And of the two, the shortness of breath and the dizziness, which was worse?

B: They were both bad but really, I guess, my breathing. Sometimes it kept me from doing much of anything.

M: OK. Let's talk about that.

Case 28

I'VE BEEN HAVING A LOT OF . . .

Dr. P: How have you been feeling, Esther?

E: Not so hot, Doctor.

P: Oh? In what way?

E: I've been having . . . a lot of . . . here [pointing to her epigastrium and right hypochondrium].

P: A lot of . . . ?

E: Yes.

P: No, I mean, what is it you have a lot of?

E: Well, it's not so bad. Not as bad as it . . . and I have some . . . here too [pointing to her flanks].

P: Uh, you have something in the middle of your belly and something in the flanks. But what is that something? Pain? Itch? What?

E: Yes.

P: Yes, what?

E: What do you mean, Doctor?

P: Let's start over again, Esther. I need to understand the symptom you have been having. You pointed to your belly and told me you had something there.

E: That's right. For a few . . .

P: A few what?

E: Well, not so long, not as long.

P: Oh dear! I need to know just what you're having there.

E: I don't know, Doctor. That's why I come here. Do you think it could be the arthritis medicine?

- What is this patient's difficulty?
- What can the doctor do?

Discussion

Although this patient is not a native English speaker, she has been living in the United States for 30 years, and I don't believe that her language problem is lack of English so much as a specific diction foible. She leaves out nouns. This person suffers from oligonounia. She doesn't need a doctor so much as a grammarian.

I think there is some sort of psychopathology behind this problem, but I don't know just what. Could it be a sort of aphasia? An anomia? Does she have a fear of naming the wrong symptom that keeps her from naming any at all? Does that same block keep her from specifying weeks or months when she tries to give a time estimate?

If anxiety is the key problem, it might yield to some understanding on the part of the doctor. Or an acknowledgment of the difficulty the doctor is having might help. Or perhaps best, a combination of the two:

P: Esther?

E: Yes, Doctor?

P: I'm having a little difficulty. I wonder if you could help me.

E: I'll try, Doctor.

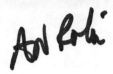

P: Well, I'm stuck when you leave out the names of what's bothering you. Can you name the symptoms? And I wonder if you're at all fearful of not getting the story told just right—if that might be hampering you.

E: Well, I surely want to help you, Doctor. What exactly do you need to know?

P: Well, for example, is it a pain you have there in your belly?

E: Not so much a pain as a, sort of, . . . hmm . . . like a . . . there!

P: Ah! Umm—is it hard for you to talk with me about it?

E: Oh no, Doctor. I always like to talk to you.

P: I see.

Unfortunately, that's about the best I've ever been able to do with this person.

Is this case too bizarre to fit in a chapter about common patient behavior? It is a one-of-a-kind in my practice. But taken as an aggregate, bizarre speech patterns add up to a big chunk of my puzzling interactions. Just listen to the next one!

Case 29

IT'S LIKE

Dr. X: Hi, Mr. Simile. How have you been doing?

S: Not so good, Doc. I've been having a lot of trouble with my kidneys.

X: What sort of trouble?

S: Well, it's like you've been sliced open and put back together. As if you had a major electrical shock and then a lot of vibration. Know what I mean?

X: Uh, no, not exactly.

S: Well, it's like you bought a new car and then discovered its muffler was out of whack. It's been going on for a while now.

X: Uh huh. Um, I'm still not sure about the symptoms . . .

S: Well, like I told you, it's like a lot of vibration. Like if you'd been eating about a bushel of green apples. See?

X: Uh, you mentioned kidneys.

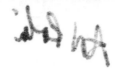

S: Yeah. Sometimes I feel that I have to go to the bathroom, and then it's like something shuts off, and then it's like there's this huge wall up there.

X: You can't pass your urine?

S: No, it passes all right. It's more like there's this machine that just isn't tuned up. Sort of like it needed a new spark plug or something. Yeah, it's like that.

X: Ah!

- Is this fellow psychotic?
- He seems to have enough nouns. Is he missing some other part of speech?

Discussion

I'm not sure he is fully sane, but I don't think he's psychotic. He does remind me a little of a schizophrenic patient who answered my mental status question, "What do a car and a truck have in common?" with "Vibration." But Dr. X assures me that this patient isn't psychotic, just has a novel way of describing his symptoms. Everything is a metaphor or a simile.

I agree that otherwise normal people, free of serious psychopathology, often seem unable to talk without bizarre circumlocutions or overformalities. Sometimes our patients sound like the police force. Everything is "alleged" and third person. "The body isn't performing its functions properly." Maybe we scare them. Maybe they think that they need to speak in a very formal "educated" style to communicate with us overeducated doctors. And some seem to love figures of speech, preferring to speak of machines they know rather than of the body they don't understand very well. Some of the problem may be a lack of basic education in human biology that leaves many people with very little understanding of human anatomy or physiology.

What can we do? The key step is to be aware of our difficulty before we get annoyed or angry about it and then to share the problem with the patient.

Our internal dialogue might be something like this:

X1: I hate this. This guy is never going to tell me anything that I can use to figure out what's wrong with him.

X2: I can imagine how frustrating it is for you. You only have a limited amount of time, and he is filling it with his mechanical analogies that don't make sense to you.

X1: Yeah. I imagine there are some clues in what he's saying, but I need a translator to figure them out.

X2: Well, maybe you ought to tell him what you need.

Then:

X: Mr. S, I'm having difficulty understanding the symptoms you are telling me about. Can you translate a little? Tell me about pain or shortness of breath or cough or nausea or whatever. Name what's happening in your body.

S: Sure, Doc. It's like there's something loose in there. Maybe a couple of parts that came unattached.

X: Oh me! I still need more help with the biological part. Maybe it would help if I asked one symptom at a time. Are you in pain?

S: Not really pain, no. It's more like a vibration.

And so it went, the doctor insisting on his version of language, the patient on his. This is a kind of power struggle that we may feel we have to win in order to give adequate medical care. Yet this man's language gives us some wonderful clues about the way he sees himself. What if we considered adopting his metaphors?

Thus:

X: Mr. S., it sounds as if you feel that your body is falling apart.

S: It sure is.

X: When you said it was like being sliced open and then put back together, I thought of being really damaged.

S: Yeah.

X: And discovering your muffler out of whack would be like discovering flaws you hadn't been aware of.

S: That's it, Doc.

X: Well, sit up on the examining table and let's see if we can find out how to tune you up.

Case 30

WHY DON'T PEOPLE ANSWER SIMPLE QUESTIONS

Dr. F: Hi, Mrs. K. How have you been doing?

K: Not so good, Doctor. I've been having a lot of pain.

F: Pain?

K: Yeah. I read that a lot of people got hepatitis this year, and I wonder if it has anything to do with . . .

F: [Interrupting] Where is the pain?

K: I didn't eat any of that Christmas pastry that that catering company made, so I don't know, but I thought I'd ask. Do you think I should take globulin shots?

F: I'm sorry, Mrs. K. I'm still confused about where the pain is.

K: Oh, up here, high up in my back.

F: And how long have you had it?

K: I think it came on when I came back from my vacation. You know the airline sent us way out of our way, through Seattle.

F: And when was that?

K: We had only been gone a week. It was right after the weather took that terrible turn for the worse. I've seen snow, but that was ridiculous.

F: Something sure is.

- What's going on here?
- Do you sometimes wonder if someone is playing a dirty trick on you, sending you patients who don't answer your simple questions with simple answers?
- Is this Mishler's life voice again?

Discussion

Strange conversations from the fourth dimension! People don't answer simple questions. They tell stories, often long stories. What's going on?

Of course many people are undisciplined conversationalists. They don't listen to the question so they don't answer it. Many of us are busy thinking of what we want to say and never listen to the other person at all.

Buie Seawell, skipper of the *Matchless*, a 44-foot sloop on which I crewed once in the mid-Atlantic, says that we should try to model our conversations more after ocean radio work. Calling a land phone from the middle of the Atlantic using ship-to-shore radio requires some specific techniques. First you identify yourself in every transmission. "Ship-to-shore, this is sailing vessel *Matchless* calling from 38 West, 41 North." Second, each participant repeats the key items from the other fellow's transmission so that he or she knows you heard correctly. "*Matchless*, 38 West, 41 North." Third, and most important, you use the magic word *over* to signal, "I am done talking and will now listen to you." Oh, that we could use *over* in our ordinary conversations! We would know just when we were responsible for listening and responding and would have a guarantee from our partner as well.

But there is more to it. Professional interviewers want specific sorts of interview data. Our clients don't know what we want, but they have desires of their own. They have stories to tell. Ordinarily stories emphasize connections, causes, and relationships. We tell about our problems as if they were stories, with many connections, and it is those connections we emphasize. The who, what, when, where, and why that we physicians yearn for are only small points in the flow of most stories. So when we ask how long the pain has been present, the patient wants to tell us who else had the pain, what might be the cause, what else is related to it. With the generosity of detail he is sharing his life with us, fleshing out his identity so that he represents himself as more than a collection of medical data. I think that's what is happening in this case. The patient is talking about linkages and causation, rather than where and how long. I think this does exemplify Mishler's "voice of the lifeworld" contrasting with the "medical voice" we use and wish our patients used [1].

This excerpt leaves unclear how the interaction had been going earlier on. Has the patient been interrupted over and over? The doctor may be contributing to the patient's storytelling drive by interrupting and thus acting uninterested in the story. Some patients consider that rude and make things worse for you.

Does it help a great deal to realize that your patient speaks a different language than you are able to hear? How does that feel to me? Usually terrible. I can sit back and enjoy the memory later, but at the time I usually feel immensely frustrated. Even my understanding of the phenomenon does not protect me from immense frustration.

5

The Database

*Ask about seat belts? Domestic violence? Are you
kidding? I've got enough to do just practicing medicine!*
                                                    Dr. Xylom

*He is the clerk of their records. He is qualified to be this
precisely because of his privilege. If the records are to be as
complete as possible—the records must be related to the
world at large, and they must include what is hidden,
even what is hidden within the protagonists themselves.*
                                                    John Berger [3]

In 1969, Morgan and Engel [31] said the medical database
obtained by interviewing the patient should include the following items:

1. Patient identification
2. Chief complaint
3. History of the present illness
4. Major past events
5. Family medical history
6. Social factors
7. Review of systems

Some medical schools in introduction to clinical medicine courses still teach such a database, but it is seriously flawed because it is incomplete. If followed, it leads to unscientific and incomplete work. As Lawrence Weed [32] has pointed out, our work seldom suffers from being too scientific, rather from the unscientific omission of critical data and the disregard of important features of our patients and their illnesses.

This database was devised to apply to a patient with a single major medical problem, but most of our patients have multiple active medical problems. As our population ages and our care of acute events improves, physicians care more and more for older patients with multiple and complex medical needs [33].

In the last few years we have become aware of other medical care needs, often because of the efforts of special interest groups: lawyers, feminists, injury prevention specialists, patient rights groups, medical ethicists, and students of doctor-patient communication. Their work has shown us the necessity of expanding our database, and primary care physicians, long devotees of historical data in patient care, realize the need for more information about our patients to work with them effectively over long time periods.

I offer the following suggestions for change (*identifies a new section of the database):

TODAY'S DATABASE

1. Patient identification
2. Chief complaint
3. Present illness
4. Other current problems*
5. Health risks*
6. Health maintenance activities*
7. Family history and genogram
8. Functional status*
9. Past medical history
10. Review of systems

11. Medical-ethical-social issues*

12. Personal character features*

Let's look at these categories one at a time.

1. Better PATIENT IDENTIFICATION. Our hospital and in-patient charts often cite the patient's age and marital status. If the patient is young, occupation may be mentioned. Seldom do we find a hint of what the past life consisted of or of what current life concerns are in the charts of our elderly patients. I suggest: age, marital status, home status (living with whom? where?), past and current occupations, and current interests and activities (how does this patient fill his/her day?).

2. CHIEF COMPLAINT, identified as the most bothersome current symptom, not the patient's self-diagnosis or the patient's idea of appropriate therapy ("right upper quadrant pain," not "gallbladder disease" or "I'm here to have my gallbladder out"). This symptom should be further defined with appropriate parameters (where, when, where else, exacerbating and relieving factors) [33, 34].

3. History of the PRESENT ILLNESS. Although we must heed the patient's story of diagnoses, treatments, and tests, we also must know the symptomatic history of the illness. The history of past doctoring (saga of medical care) will not be enough.

*4. OTHER CURRENT ACTIVE PROBLEMS. Studies show that our patients have an average of three major active problems. We know that failure to elicit these active problems early in the history provokes several bothersome interview syndromes including "a full review of systems" and the "by the way, doctor . . ." syndrome. If elicited at this stage of the history, the other current active problems will fall easily into a problem-oriented listing. In fact, the problem first described by our patient may well not be his or her most important one, either in our eyes or in the patient's.

If left to be uncovered during the review of systems, these problems will not be ordered by patient priority and we often will not know if they are current or active or significantly bothersome. So we need to ask at this stage of the history, "What else is troubling you?" "What other current active major problems do you have?" "Besides this first problem (as listed in the present illness), what other problems are you having?" And somewhere we need to ask just what the patient most wanted to accomplish by this visit [35].

*5. HEALTH HAZARDS. Some of these have traditionally been hidden in the "social" section of the history [36]. We need to detail them fully and may need subschemata to do so. Topics that need investigation and inclusion in the health hazard section include alcohol intake, including the CAGE questions [37]; cigarette use; over-the-counter and street drug use; prescription medication; use/nonuse of seat belts in vehicles; motorcycles and bicycles and concomitant nonuse of helmets; exposure to other work and domestic injury hazards, especially those of domestic violence—the key question may be "Are you now or have you been in the past living in fear of someone's violence?" [24]; sedentary lifestyle; diet, including an estimate of caloric intake and carbohydrate, fat, and protein breakdown; sexual risks [38, 39]; allergies to drugs; and so on.

*6. HEALTH MAINTENANCE ACTIVITIES. This is the other side of the previous category: cancer self-checking activities, use of ancillary tests such as mammograms and Pap smears [40], exercise programs, dietary limitations, and so on.

7. FAMILY GENOGRAM. We are first concerned with who is who in the family, what their functional relationship is with the patient, and how close and available they are for support purposes. We are more concerned with family dynamics than family illnesses. Then we must inquire about the real familial disorders—smoking, drinking, obesity, suicide, violence—more than diseases that we know to have faint family linkages. Finally, we must know if any-

one in the family has anything like what the patient has or the patient thinks he or she might have [41].

*8. FUNCTIONAL ABILITIES. Especially with our older patients and those hampered by chronic diseases, we must know what they can and can't do [42]. Can they dress themselves? Walk? Use the toilet? Transfer independently? Feed themselves? Do they get lost or mixed up when out of the house? Are they having trouble with function in any sphere?

9. MAJOR PAST EVENTS: illnesses, operations, and hospitalizations.

10. REVIEW OF SYSTEMS (should be empty of really important problems by now) [43].

*11. MEDICAL-SOCIAL-ETHICAL ISSUES [44, 45]: Who is the responsible agent? Have decisions been made for future care (living will, power of attorney, DNR status)? Who is to be contacted if the patient becomes ill and is unable to inform us? What are the present living arrangements, and what changes are contemplated?

*12. CHARACTER FEATURES: What sort of person is this [46]? Osler's key to understanding: "It is more important to know what sort of a person this disease has than to know what sort of a disease this person has." Since much of medicine consists of an ongoing therapeutic relationship, an understanding of the patient's character is critical. Much of this may be hard for the patient to tell you, but simple features may be available even early on: Do you prefer to take medicines or wait out an illness if the choice is close? What sort of treatment do you prefer? What most aggravates you?

This is a massive expansion of our usual database. We need not explore each area at every visit, nor can we explore all of them on a first visit, but we can accumulate the data as we care for the patient. These are valid areas for medical attention, and changes in status will affect the quality of care we can provide. It is not adequate for a patient followed in one of our clinics to have no genogram detailed after three years of visits. We cannot be proud of a patient's care when the existence of domestic violence is revealed only after years of caring for the patient. We should expect an initial encounter to include patient identification, present illness, and other active concerns in all but the most emergent situations. Health hazards should be our next area of concern.

A logistic problem: Should the database reside in a fixed place in the patient's medical record? If so, entries will need to be dated as they are first noted and placed in the chart. And some entries will need to change over time (family members die, the patient adopts a healthier lifestyle, etc.). As an alternative, the database may be entered chronologically in progress notes. An index or table of contents then should be found at the front of the chart. Thus, under "Genogram," for example, there might be several dates entered as changes occur.

It is also clear that much of these data can be obtained by patients' filling out questionnaires and by ancillary personnel. Computerized charting may solve many of our logistic problems. Physician time may be increased by such an expanded database, but physicians are not the only people who can obtain the data.

An improved, more thorough database would lead to improved, more thorough medical care. I am confident that many of the flaws of our current care arise from our lack of basic knowledge about patients' lives.

Case 31

THE BURNING IN MY STOMACH

The patient was an 80-year-old man who entered the hospital for removal of an infected hip prosthesis. His admission history and physical examination were done by his orthopedist, who admitted that he was brief with the review of systems, mostly asking if the patient had any additional problems. The patient was then seen in consultation by a cardiologist, who focused on his past history of angina and myocardial infarction and his current frequent premature ventricular beats. He was also seen by a pulmonologist, who focused on his chronic obstructive lung disease. Prior to admission to the hospital, the patient had been taking an inhaled beta-agonist bronchodilator, quinidine, and an occasional aspirin.

The operation went well, and the patient seemed to be recovering nicely until four days after surgery when he suddenly began to vomit great quantities of blood. He had been treated postoperatively with Coumadin to maintain his prothrombin time between 16 and 18 seconds. A gastroenterologist was asked to see the patient. On endoscopy, he found a bleeding duodenal ulcer and was able to cauterize it partially. A general internist was asked to see the patient "to pull all his assorted parts back together." He stopped the Coumadin and treated the patient with fresh frozen plasma. The patient was transfused with red blood cells, and a total of eight units was needed before bleeding stopped. The general internist's conversation with the patient included this fragment:

Dr X: Prior to this episode, have you had any belly symptoms?
Mr A: Nope. I've always had an iron stomach.
X: No heartburn? Indigestion? Stomach pain?
A: Nope.
X: And your medicines were the bronchodilator, the quinidine, and one aspirin a day?
A: That's it, Doc. Just my breathing medicine and those two others.
X: Any other medicines? Headache pills? Anything for arthritis or aches or pains?
A: Nope.
X: Tums or Rolaids? Antacids?
A: Nope.
X: Nothing, then, but what you told us. No other potions or pills?
A: Nope. Except for the Pepto-Bismol.
X: Pepto-Bismol?
A: Yeah. I take it for the burning in my stomach.
X: Burning in your stomach?
A: Yeah, right here [pointing to his epigastrium].

X: Ah! And how much Pepto-Bismol do you have to take?
A: Not much, Doc. Maybe about six swigs a day.

- If this doctor had stopped pressing the patient about medicines one step earlier, the history of ulcer pain and ulcer therapy wouldn't have appeared. How are we to know when to stop asking?

- If this doctor had seen the patient preoperatively, would he have turned up this history? Would he have learned enough to preclude treatment of an active duodenal ulcer with anticoagulants?

- Why is this patient so reticent about his belly symptoms? Do we need to ask about pain with the precise wording the patient uses ("burning in the stomach")?

- What do you think of doing a review of systems by asking if there are any other active problems?

Discussion

It is amazing that people do not consider their over-the-counter remedies to be medicines. Sometimes they fail to realize that vitamins, analgesics, birth control pills, or any chronically taken medications should be counted and reported to the doctor. One rule of thumb for asking important questions is to ask anything you really care about three times, in three different ways. So it is reasonable to ask about medications several times and with several different phrasings. Even then, I find it easy to miss important data. The same reticence to provide data about medications seems to crop up again in this patient's inability to mention his abdominal pain until the magic words "burning in the belly" are used. This overspecificity seems too much for any doctor to cope with, and I believe the root cause in this patient is an organic brain syndrome. His thinker isn't working right.

Sometimes our subspecialists do seem overfocused, attending mostly to the problems they consider to fall in their own bailiwicks. Unless the patient is cared for by every subspecialist in the book, important areas might go unnoticed. This case provides a good argument for the role of a generalist in patient care. It might be that a generalist would have tumbled to the presence of chronic belly pain or to the self-therapy with antacids prior to surgery. But it would have been a toss-up even then.

The review of systems is a big headache to me. I think we overemphasize it in medical school and residency. Use of an extensive series of questions undermines formation of a good doctor-patient relationship by encouraging a high-control style and suppressing the patient's voluntary utterances. A patient subjected to such questioning often perceives his interlocutor as "a doctor who didn't want to listen to me." I prefer to use "ROS-emptying questions" such as "Is there anything else troubling you?" or "Any other current active problems?" Then I tend to do a very abbreviated review of systems, trusting my emptying devices to have picked up anything that is current, active, and important. However my approach may not be enough. Mitchell et al. [43] recently studied the yield of a screening review of systems with special emphasis on cardiopulmonary and gastrointestinal questions. Of 207 patients with no known GI disease, they found 45 who gave a total of 71 positive answers to their screening GI questions and made 22 new GI diagnoses in these 207 patients. It may be that even after efforts to empty the review of systems, we will pick up a sizable number of disorders by a careful and thorough questioning protocol. That is the bad news. We may still need that ROS.

In this patient, I might well have failed to press further for gastrointestinal symptoms when they were initially denied. Of course, once the gastrointestinal bleeding was identified, it makes sense to ask any related question one can think of, maybe even "Do you have burning in your stomach?"

Case 32

CHICKEN HAWK

JS: Doc, I've got a new problem. I've got these sores on my genitals.
Dr. Xylom: I see. Tell me more.

JS: Not much to tell. I just noticed them this weekend, two days ago. They sting and burn some, but that's all.

X: I see. Are you sexually active, John?

JS: Yeah, I am. Last time was a couple of weeks ago.

X: Uh huh. And are you active mostly with women or men?

JS: Well, both, I guess. Mostly I'm a chicken hawk.

X: What? What's that?

JS: Oh Jesus! Doc, you know.

X: No, I don't. What's a chicken hawk?

JS: Oh shit! [Gets up and paces about in the examining room.] Can you just look at the sores? I don't have much time.

X: OK. Let's see.

The patient drops his trousers and shorts. The doctor dons a glove and examines the groin, genitalia, and then the perianal area.

X: I see. You have a little cluster of tiny ulcers on the shaft of your penis. That's what you're talking about?

JS: Yeah.

X: Well, almost surely herpes simplex. We can get a culture on it and start you taking some acyclovir. That ought to help.

JS: OK, doc. That's what I thought it was. Just wanted your opinion. Do I take these pills five times a day? I have a friend who has it, and that's how he takes them.

X: Yes, that's right. If you follow the prescription you should have a shorter course of this first outbreak. It might well recur though.

JS: I know all that, Doc. I'll let you know if it recurs.

- How do you approach the task of acquiring a sexual history?

- What do you do if you don't understand the patient's terminology in this delicate area?

Discussion

This doctor started out fairly well, inquiring about sexual orientation; however he let his patient escape from the questions when the patient became uncomfortable. The doctor was feeling foolish, he later said, about his ignorance of contemporary sexual terms. Imagine how he would have felt if he realized that his patient was trying to tell him that he was bisexual and that his usual partners were young boys! The patient surely needed to discuss this issue with his doctor, but the doctor's lack of knowledge of the term dissuaded him from further conversation. What could the doctor have done?

I think the best course would be to note the patient's consternation, interpret it as evidence of the patient's strong feelings about what he was trying to say, and help him with the explanation. Instead, this doctor was busy thinking of his own feelings, mostly those of embarrassment about ignorance and discomfort talking about sexual issues.

The doctor could have said:

X: I see that this is an important issue but hard to talk about. I'm pretty ignorant about the variety of sexual arrangements, but I promise not to be judgmental and not to run away.

What then? Maybe the patient could have explained just what a chicken hawk is, just what his sexual activity consisted of.

After this doctor fainted, recovered, picked himself up, and thought about the description, perhaps they could have gone on to a useful therapeutic discussion, including an exploration of the morality of having sex with young boys. After all, sex with young boys or girls is not a matter we can address without considering moral values. The patient's behavior may well constitute child abuse, and if so, it is a crime. I suspect that the patient knows this and that his naming his sexual practice was an attempt to engage with someone he trusted and respected—his physician—in a discussion about it. This is a magnificent opportunity to use our humane skills, accepting the patient while challenging his behavior. Exploring the patient's hesitance about explaining his sexual practices, probing to see if he acknowledges that his behavior is criminal and abusive, and voicing concern about what the patient is doing are all within the scope of our duties as caregivers. To an imagined, "But I'm not a policeman . . ." my reply is that police are our last line of response to hurtful behaviors. Doctors, like everyone else, are neighbors, friends, and citizens, and we have a duty to our community to respond when we see something wrong going on. But we also have an enormously powerful position with our patients and a real chance to help them change behavior without punitive action.

Finally, even about the physical disease, the herpes simplex eruption, the doctor needs to do some contact investigation or report the case to the state health system for such investigation, and he shouldn't assume that his patient has a good understanding of the disease or of its therapy until he has explained more.

Case 33

BIGMOUTH

Dr. A recently installed Bigmouth, a program to handle phone messages, in his office computer. The program answers the phone evenings and weekends, records the message, and summons Dr. A by ringing his pager. Tuesday evening he was paged and found this message in his voice mail:

S: Dr. A, this is Susan. I'm at a pay phone and I have to leave, so you can't call me back, but I need to talk to you. Can you please call me tomorrow after 4:30? I'm having a terrible time at work. They are probably going to fire me. I need something for my nerves.

The next day, Dr. A made several attempts to call Susan before and after 4:30. There was no answer at her home phone. Thursday morning, as soon as the office was open but an hour before Dr. A was to arrive, the patient called again and talked with Dr. A's assistant, Pamela.

S: This is Susan. I need to talk to Dr. A. I'm so upset. I'm having a terrible time at work. I need him to give me something for my nerves.

P: What sort of trouble are you having?

S: I'm just upset. They are treating me terribly. I gave notice to quit in June, and then they just went and fired me. They gave me one-week notice. I can't sleep, and I'm terribly upset.

P: Can you come in to talk with the doctor? I'm sure he'd want to see you, and we would make a time for you.

S: No, I can't today. And he can't call me at work. I'll try to call him again tonight. I'm so upset, I think I'm going to kill my boss.

P: Wait, Susan. Tell me a number where we can reach you.

S: No, I can't. I gotta go now. I'll call later.

P: No, wait, Susan . . . [phone now dead].

Pamela carefully detailed this conversation in the patient's chart. When Dr. A arrived at the office 20 minutes later, he found the patient's chart on his desk with a note saying, "Susan called. She says she is very upset and thinks she is going to kill her boss. She will call back later."

- What should Dr. A do?
- What will happen if Dr. A calls the police?
- What will happen if Susan shoots her boss?

Discussion

Dr. A suspects that Susan is distraught but not homicidal. However, he had only seen her twice in the past and does not think that he knows her capabilities. Not comfortable with ignoring her obvious pleas for help, he wonders if it might be reasonable to wait until she gets in touch with him again.

Dr. A might have felt less anxious if Pamela hadn't so scrupulously detailed her conversation with Susan in the chart. If Pamela had only mentioned it to him, Dr. A might have been able to minimize the threat and perhaps would have let his intuition guide his actions. He would have waited for her next call.

Unfortunately that could be too late, perhaps too late to

help Susan and possibly too late to help her boss. The courts have told us that we are obliged to act when a patient says that he or she might be contemplating a violent act on another person. We must inform the police and through them, the potential victim. Most often cited is the case of *Tarasoff* v. *Board of Regents of the University of California.* The California Supreme Court ruled that a therapist had a paramount duty to warn a potential victim.

It is very possible that Susan is not in severe distress and even more likely that she is neither suicidal nor homicidal. She would probably be unhappy if the police appeared at her door, and the police may refuse to intervene. Whatever we do is likely to be too much or too little. Dr. A decided to wait.

In this case, the patient finally made an effective connection with her doctor the next day. She was anxious and depressed, even somewhat paranoid, but neither suicidal nor homicidal. She had not intended her comment to be taken literally. She insisted that she had no weapon and had no intention of harming her ex-boss. Eventually she found a new job, recovered from her distressing experiences, and went on with her life.

This book focuses on medical conversations, but this case presents NO CONVERSATION between doctor and patient. A rarity? Not so! How often we now return urgent telephone calls to find ourselves talking to an answering machine. What a mess! Then what are our medical and legal obligations? Can we consider a message we leave on a machine to be effective communication? Surely not. So how can we be happy with Bigmouth as our representative? I expect we all will be hearing more on this sort of subject from the courts in the future.

Case 34

TELL ME ABOUT YOURSELF

The physician had just attended a workshop on doctor-patient communication. He was full of new ideas and eager to try them out. One suggestion made at the workshop had been to spend a little time "getting to know the patient" before digging into the medical concerns. Dr. Xylom tried it out.

X: Mrs. A, before we get to the medical concerns, how about telling me about yourself.

A: OK. I used to consult Dr. Y, but my insurance changed and I had to find another doctor. I've been having a lot of trouble with my bursitis, and I think that maybe I've got that thing in my knees, chondromalitis. I've had two back operations and a hysterectomy. Is that what you wanted to know?

X: Umm, I sort of thought maybe you could tell me more about yourself as a person, not just your medical history.

A: OK. Like what?

X: Well, uh, just sort of a personal description, uh.

A: Like what I like to do? Or where I'm from?

X: Yeah, that would be OK.

A: Well, I'm from Detroit, but I've lived out here since 1954. I guess that I like the usual things, visiting and going out with my friends, and mostly I work and stay home.

X: Yes?

A: That's it. What else do you want to know?

X: Oh gosh, I don't know. Maybe you ought to tell me what brought you to me today.

- Dr. X says that he thought it would be easy to get his patient to tell about herself, and now he finds that he is stuck. Any suggestions?

- If you had to set up a checklist of important items to cover to get an idea of "just what sort of a person this is," what would you include?

Discussion

I have read that people are eager to talk about themselves. Everyone has his own story, supposedly, and wants to tell it. Maybe so, but I too have found patients tongue-tied when I asked them to tell me about themselves. Some leap in and enjoy the opportunity. Others are stuck, perhaps shy, perhaps just have never formulated a life story.

If the patient is stuck, the easiest approach is first to elicit the usual life milestones and defining markers. Married or single? Significant other? Children? Where does she live and with whom? Work? How does she mostly spend her time? What are her other major interests and concerns? Where was she from, and where did she grow up and go to school? Previous jobs? Previous marriages? Friends? Pets? Who is available to her for support? We could imagine a protocol for all this just as we think of the protocol of the review of systems.

Perhaps more important, what sort of person does she seem to be? Is she stoical or more likely to call for help? Optimistic or pessimistic? Straightforward or oblique? Careful and methodical or more disorganized? Does she become more calm in emergencies or more agitated? How does she feel about collaborating with a physician? Is she responsible or careless of her health?

Unless the case is an emergency, you can elicit the patient's social history as you obtain her medical history, formulating an overall impression of character as a result of the way she reports. As you continue to work with the patient, these data will be invaluable in recruiting her cooperation and interpreting her responses. I do not believe that the social inquiry is best delayed to the end of the history. I prefer to dedicate a little bit of time early on to this purpose. Greg Carroll suggests asking for the patient's permission and understanding first: "I like to get to know some personal background from patients before we get into your illness history because I feel that knowing you as a person is very important to my function as a doctor. How does that sound to you?"

Case 35

IT'S HARD NOT TO SMOKE

Ms. Puff appeared at the emergency department complaining of nightly episodes of tremulousness and palpitations. The spells lasted 30 to 60 minutes and were quite frightening. She was a long-term smoker and suffered with dyspnea but little cough. The emergency department doctor called Dr. Xylom.

Dr. Y: Dr. X? This is Y here. I have a patient who has no doctor and needs to come into the hospital. She's got bad COPD, but what will convince you to admit her is her chest x-ray. She's got a big left hilar mass.

X: Hmm. That might be the one reason not to admit her. If she has a big cancer and bad COPD, we probably have little to offer. But I'll be over and take a look at her in about 20 minutes. OK?

The patient was admitted, placed on an ECG monitor, and given various tests. Her chest CT showed large pulmonary arteries; the left hilar mass wasn't a tumor after all. However, she also had an aneurysm of the descending aorta and what appeared to be a benign tumor of the right adrenal gland. We spent several days looking for functional adrenal abnormalities—none were discovered—and considering surgery that neither she nor a vascular surgeon thought a good idea. She had no further symptoms of tremulousness or palpitations. She was treated with transdermal nicotine patches and a low-dose beta blocker. She went home, reassured that no cancer had been found, and promised to stop smoking and to keep a follow-up appointment at Dr. X's office.

Three weeks later, having missed her office appointment, she returned to the emergency department complaining of nocturnal tremulousness and palpitations. The ED physician called Dr. X:

Dr. Z: What will really convince you to admit her is her chest x-ray. I think the mediastinum is wider. Her aneurysm is getting worse.

The next day, Dr. X again interviewed Ms. Puff.

X: How have you been doing with the smoking?
P: Not so good, Doctor. I'm still smoking. But I've cut down.
X: Oh? How much are you smoking now?

P: About a pack a day. But lots of time I don't smoke—the cigarette just sits in its ashtray.

X: Uh huh? That sounds like about the amount you told me you were smoking when you were here last month.

P: Yeah, about that. It's hard to quit though. It's hard not to smoke when you have a cup of coffee in your hand.

X: Coffee? Oh! I never asked you about coffee. How many cups do you drink each day?

P: I can't even guess that, Doctor. I don't know about cups. I have a pot going all day. I drink pots.

X: Pots, eh? If you tried a guess, how many cups do you drink in a day? Ten?

P: Oh no, not ten. At least twice that many.

X: And you are having spells at night with palpitations and tremulousness?

P: Yeah. [Smiling] I wondered if the coffee had anything to do with it.

Dr. X reviewed her chest x-ray with a radiologist. They both thought it entirely unchanged from the prior films done a month before. Her mediastinum had not widened.

Now understanding how his patient's symptoms had vanished on the prior admission, a hospital stay that didn't include double-digit coffee cupping, Dr. X discharged her from the hospital with a prescription for nicotine patches, beta blockers, and a promise to avoid cigarettes and coffee. She was to be seen in the office in a week.

Three weeks later, again having missed her office appointment, Ms. P arrived at the emergency department at 5 A.M., brought in by ambulance. She had awakened at 3 A.M. with "a ton of bricks on my chest," accompanied by tremulousness and diaphoresis. Two nitroglycerin tablets administered in the ambulance gave her relief. She felt fine when the ED doctor interviewed her. He called Dr. X.

Dr. W: I think she has a worrisome story. But what will really convince you is her ECG. She has hyperacute T waves.

X: OK. Put her upstairs on a monitor bed, please, and notify the medical house staff. I'll see her in an hour or two.

When Dr. X saw Ms. P, she was feeling "fine." She admitted to smoking three cigarettes a day but carried a strong tobacco aroma with her. She said that she was down to 12 cups of coffee a day.

The cardiogram was, of course, unchanged from prior tracings, showing some minimal right ventricular enlargement but no T wave changes, specifically no "hyperacute T waves." The physical examination was unchanged from prior visits. She had nearly absent breath sounds throughout her lungs. Twenty-four hours of monitoring, enzyme determinations, and repeat ECGs disclosed no abnormality.

- What now?
- Do you always ask about coffee? Would this doctor have fewer miraculous coups if he would just take a more thorough history?
- What about all the "This should convince you" comments from the emergency department?

Discussion

"What now?" is really a puzzler. The damage is mostly already done. Ms. P has far advanced emphysema and probably considerable coronary artery disease as well. Even if she does stop smoking, she may not be around much longer. Still, we are often surprised, and I think it is fair to try to help her discontinue the cigarettes. It won't be easy. For one thing, she lives in an apartment building with many friendly neighbors, all of whom smoke and drink many cups of coffee as they visit each other daily. The cigarettes and the coffee are part of her social milieu, and that social world is very important to her. Prochaska et al. [47] suggest that we identify the patient's stage in coming to grips with her smoking. Does she deny its health danger and want no discussion or help with smoking? Has she advanced to recognize the hazard but still not readiness to stop? Is she ready to stop, only lacking a firm date? Has she decided when to stop smoking and thus is accessible to our help with nicotine patches or stop-smoking groups? If we don't know where she is, we can't very well help to move her to the next stage.

An incomplete history seems unavoidable. Any admission history/physical examination is bound to be incomplete. For example, do you review cancer screening behavior? Health hazards such as nonuse of seat belts, existence of domestic violence, presence of handguns at the home? Medical ethical issues such as living wills, durable power of attorney for medical decision making, or other desires for care and noncare if the patient cannot make her wishes known? In fact, a complete database that will satisfy medical ethicists, experts in domestic violence, legal demands, cancer screening experts, family therapists, and so on might take hours. We are never that complete. We are never thorough enough. There will always be amazing discoveries, surprises, and sudden disclosures. The best strategy may be to establish an atmosphere that is conducive to just these sorts of disclosures. If we can never be thorough enough, perhaps we can be open to miraculous surprise.

The emergency department seems wedded to technology. If you are a bit cynical, you might suspect that we get whatever we pay for and currently are mostly paying for technology. But it does tickle my funny bone that the three declarations of "What will convince you" in this case were all erroneous. When in doubt, I still think the history and the physical examination have the best yield. Of course, we have to ask about those pots of coffee.

Case 36

I'VE NEVER TOLD ANYONE

Dr. X's patient, Mary Anne, was well known to him. A 40-year-old woman who had many past hospitalizations for psychosis, she seemed to be doing better except for recurrent bouts of acute bronchitis. Another such bout brought her back to the office.

X: Hello, Mary Anne. I see you're here today because of more coughing.

MA: Yes, Doctor. I've got it again. Coughing up green stuff again.
X: Ah! Let's see. I treated you with Ceftin a month ago.
MA: Yes, Doctor.
X: And are you still smoking?
MA: Oh, yes, Doctor; I'm afraid I am. I'm so embarrassed.
X: So no surprise that you've got bronchitis again, is it? How're you ever going to get rid of it if you don't stop?
MA: Oh, Doctor, please don't be angry with me.
X: Well, this is ridiculous. You keep coming back with these lung infections!
MA: Yes, Doctor.

[Pause.]

X: Mary Anne, I wonder. Have you ever been abused?
MA: Not now, Doctor. But yes, when I was younger.
X: Physical abuse? Sexual?
MA: Well, both, Doctor. The really hard part was the sexual abuse. I've never told anyone before.

She then proceeded to tell her story of familial incest and mistreatment. Most of the story had never been told before, even with several psychiatric hospitalizations and interviews by many therapists.

- What happened to Dr. X during the pause?
- What do you include in your routine history under the category of "health hazards"?
- How do you approach the issues of domestic violence and sexual abuse?
- Do you ask your male patients of their past history of abuse? As victims? As perpetrators?

Discussion

Dr. X says that he suddenly felt himself to be acting in an abusive way when he was haranguing MA about her smoking. It gave him pause, and he took the opportunity to reflect a moment. That led him to wonder about MA's past history and to ask the simple question. Dr. X had recently read Judith Herman's book, *Trauma and Recovery* [24]. He was impressed with Herman's description of the correlation between women's self-abusive behavior and a history of rape, incest, and prolonged abusive familial relationships. It prompted him to explore these issues with MA.

Perhaps the patient too sensed a replication of painful childhood experiences as her doctor browbeat her about smoking. Perhaps she sensed a parallel with her earlier abusive experiences. She surely seemed ready to talk when asked.

How to ask about abuse? I like Herman's questions: "Are you now living in fear of someone's violence? Have you in the past?" And we can ask, "Have you been a victim of sexual abuse? Is it still going on?" I think these belong in every history along with questions about the presence of guns in the home, use or nonuse of automobile seat belts, use or nonuse of motorcycle and bicycle helmets, and exercise patterns.

And I think we miss something important if we don't address domestic violence with our male patients. It's true that 95% of the victims of domestic abuse are female. But 95% of the perpetrators are male. We could ask the men we care for if they are troubled by excessive anger or anger out of control. As with the CAGE queries about alcoholism, we could ask, "Have you ever done anything when you were angry that you later felt sorry for?" We can ask about family arguments. Everyone has them. "When you and your wife argue, what happens? Does anyone get hit?" If we don't ask these sorts of questions, we won't hear the answers. We need to hear them to help our patients, male and female.

Finally, a reminder. I locate this case in the Database chapter. It fits here. But it could just as easily be approached with other techniques, that of discovering meaning, for example. There are many routes to the same end.

6

The Doctor Did It

My doctor doesn't listen to me.

Patient of Dr. Xylom

The qualities that best exemplify the characteristics of the ideal physician: He is constantly observant, uses a systematic approach, knows and understands basic principles, uses reason in all his actions, is aware of the limitations of his own knowledge and of knowledge in general, respects the information that comes from the patient, and is a perpetual student.

W. L. Morgan, Jr. and G. L. Engel [31]

Although we blame the patient for most of our problems, it turns out that many of the difficult interviews we experience or observe are made difficult by specific actions of the physician. The doctor is one of the two actors in a doctor-patient interchange and is often the source of the difficulty. That shouldn't surprise us, but there has been a relative paucity of studies of flawed doctor technique compared to the plethora of articles about difficult patients in the medical literature [10, 48].

CONTROL FREAKS

The doctor's use of control may seem too simple a problem to warrant a section all of its own. However I know no problem as disabling for the doctor-patient interaction, none so ubiquitous, and no other that seems so clearly to be a product of our system of medical education. Our doctors get worse as they proceed through the training programs. Students tend not to overcontrol the interview, but our graduating senior residents have perfected the technique. I hypothesize that the resident learns medicine by floating through subspecialty rotations where he learns clusters of specific questions. By the end of his residency, the doctor has 20 questions from cardiology, 20 from gastroenterology, and so on, perhaps a sum of 200 important questions to have answered. Many residents seem to think that a good interview is an immense review of systems conducted with a huge battery of yes-no questions, a process that is inhumane, is time costly, and fails to prioritize.

Patients recognize the problem right away. They say, "He's probably a good doctor, but he doesn't listen to me." Or, "He's arrogant. I wouldn't recommend him."

What I call a high-control style can be recognized by weighing the conversation. The doctor's comments outnumber the patient's. Ideally, in a medical interview, the doctor would state what he needs to know and then would get out of the way of the patient. There would be a lot more patient words than doctor words. But a high-control doctor doesn't give his patient much room to talk. The doctor assaults the patient with a barrage of questions that allow increasingly narrow answers. Pretty soon the patient is answering with simple yes and no replies.

ASYMPTOMATIC HISTORY

If we view physician communication styles as a continuum of behaviors, the style opposite high control is passivity. The doctor who listens passively will usually elicit an asymptomatic history. He sits by while the patient provides diagnoses, theories of causation, and suggestions of further therapeutic steps but fails to tell his symptoms. The passive doctor may even choose to hear nonsymptom material instead of symptoms:

Dr. X: What sort of trouble were you having?
Patient A: Well, I have heart trouble, and this week I've been feeling dizzy.
X: Tell me about the heart trouble.

Of course I commiserate with Dr. X. Who wants to hear another story of dizziness? Still, that's the symptom that this patient has provided and the one that we have to explore. Asking about the heart trouble is following the patient's diagnosis instead of the symptom. That's a no-no. I think of this patient as an old radio with two knobs. One knob is labeled "signal" and the other "noise." Asking about the heart disease amounts to turning up the volume on the noise knob.

This behavior is characteristic of neophytes. Student interviewers are often shy about directing the interview where they have to move it and often don't know where it has to go anyway, so they tend to accept the patient's story, whatever it is. It saddens me that the end product of our residency training programs is too often a high-pressure doctor. The resident gives up one flawed style only to adopt another.

I don't think these two opposite syndromes are so ubiquitous by accident. I credit a real dilemma that is at the heart of medical interviewing. Mishler might say that we have to be able to hear the story both in the language of the life world and in the language of medicine. Indeed, we have the joint challenge of directing the patient to tell a symptomatic history and of staying out of his way. That isn't easy. If it were, we would all do it all the time.

Case 37

GOSH!

L: Hello, Ms. F. I'm Dr. L. I'm the intern working on this ward. I need to talk with you and ask you some questions.
F: OK.

L: Well, maybe you can start by telling me what brought you to the hospital.

F: I was vomiting for a week. I'm 67 and that's hard on me. I got dizzy and nauseated first; that had been going on for three weeks. And my sugars were high.

L: How long were you sick?

F: It started about three weeks ago. I was . . .

L: Anything to go with the nausea? Did you have headaches?

F: I almost passed out. Once in the car, in the parking lot.

L: Gosh!

F: I did pass out once.

L: You have diabetes? When did you get it? How old were you?

F: That was about 15 years ago.

L: Do you take insulin?

F: Yes, I . . .

L: How much insulin?

F: Well, I usually take fifteen units of U100 . . .

L: Who is your doctor?

F: Dr. A.

L: OK. Any other medicines?

F: Oh yes. Lots. I take Procardia and Vasotec and Synthroid and Premarin and aspirin . . .

L: Why the Procardia?

F: High blood pressure. I have high blood pressure.

L: Do you have problems with your heart? Chest pain?

F: I had one here. It was nothing though. They said it was OK.

L: OK. Any family diseases?

- What do you think of "Gosh!"?
- What is the theme of this interview?

Discussion

I like the "gosh!" better than the rest of the interview.

Dr. L has a lovely smile and radiates enthusiasm and good cheer to her patients. They like her immediately. That rapport helps compensate for a high-pressure interview style that, in itself, is very destructive.

Dr. L uses questions as her only interview device. In addition, she doesn't let the patient answer them before she is in there with another question. Her questioning is rather narrow—"Do you take insulin?" instead of "How do you treat the diabetes?" And the questions constitute no coherent interview scheme.

What could Dr. L do to improve her technique? Most of all, give the patient room to talk. Don't be afraid of a little silence. Beckman and Frankel [49] studied outpatient interviews and found that doctors in their sample allowed their patients to talk an average of 18 seconds before interrupting. That's not enough, and Dr. L doesn't even allow 18 seconds. She could give her patient a whole minute or even more to tell the story of the present illness, only using facilitatory nods and hums to help her along. She could start by stating the task: "I need you to tell me about this trouble you have been having, especially the symptoms that have been bothering you." And then she could stop talking, stay out of the patient's way, and let the story come forth. Even later, with simpler questions, Dr. L should allow enough time for the patient to finish her answers. That necessary time extends past the point where the patient stops talking. You have to let the patient think a bit and perhaps add to her answer.

Next, this doctor could try a couple of other devices besides questions. She could ask for help. "I need you to tell me about the diabetes" or "I need you to tell me about any other medical problems you're having." She might try some one-word inquiries: "Diabetes?"

I prefer the interview to begin with a minute or two devoted to identifying the patient before we get into the illness. It helps form an alliance and helps place the medical problems in context. Maybe not much, just the patient's age and situation in life, work and family, major activities and concerns.

Time in the medical interview is like money in the bank. Early investment leads to great savings. The doctor often thinks she has to rush to save time and that questions help. Not so! Questions fill up the time with doctor talk when what we need is to hear the patient.

What about the "Gosh!"? Why do I like it so much? I think

it is shorthand, standing for a longer communication, something like: "I heard what you said and have been thinking about how it must feel for you, and I really understand the weight of the moment." It is an empathic utterance and carries the message: "I am with you."

Case 38

CHEST THUMP

Dr. M: I'm glad to meet you, Mr. L. Perhaps I can sit here by your bed, and then you can tell me about the problems you've been having. These doctors are the rest of our ward teaching team, and they're going to listen in to our conversation.

L: That's fine, Doctor. I used to teach interviewing for an insurance company, so I'm used to it.

M: OK. What sort of troubles have you been having?

L: I was fine until 4:45 A.M. on Monday. Then suddenly I had a "woosh" and my bowels went. Pure blood. All black. I had about five of them like that.

M: [nodding.]

L: And there was that sour pain. But mostly it was just the black bowels that got me in here.

M: What do you mean, "sour pain?"

L: Kind of here [points to the epigastrium], just a sour pain.

M: Had that before?

L: Well, a couple of years ago I had some, and I was pretty sure that my heart had stopped. So I hit myself here [demonstrating by thumping his chest over the precordium] a couple of times. Then I went across the street to my neighbor who is a chiropractor. He said I had a hiatal hernia, and he manipulated me pretty roughly. It hurt like hell, but it did the trick, and I haven't had that pain since.

M: Is that right!

L: But Sunday I had some of that pain again in the pit of my stomach.

M: OK. Let me see if I've got the story right. You had that pain on Sunday . . .

L: Maybe a little bit the day before.

M: Uh huh. And then you started having black stools. Any other symptoms?

L: I was pretty dizzy a couple of times. I saw stars there. Then I came to the hospital and saw Dr. K. He put me on oxygen for two days.

M: So what else has happened?

L: They put this thing down my throat. I had a terrific dry throat. You know I had TB in the 40s. They used to put a big tube down my throat every morning when I was at Lutheran in 1942. I hated that. Those days you had to swallow a big tube. Not like now.

M: Any other tests?

L: Well they found a stomach ulcer. Then, of course, I've got a heart problem. That's why they give me the Vasotec.

M: What sort of heart problem?

L: Emphysema. And I never smoked. But I used to travel a lot. I've driven over a million miles, I guess. And as much on trains and planes. And you got exposed to a lot of smoke in those days. Everyone else smoked.

M: That's a lot of miles.

L: Yeah. There was a guy in the office who kept coughing. That was before I came down with tuberculosis. Then they took him away. There were a lot of smokers too. I worked at Boeing during World War II as an engineer and everyone smoked.

M: Sounds like quite a bit of exposure to smoking.

L: Yes. And I had pneumonia when I was about nine. I was out of my head. The doctor put me up on the kitchen table and gave me ether and cut open my chest. I died and came back. I had one of those "near death" experiences. They didn't believe me at first, but I did.

M: Huh. Have you any other heart problems? Heart attacks? Chest pain?

L: Just my gallbladder. I had pain once for six hours. I thought it was my heart, but they told me it was the gallbladder.

M: Did you ever have a heart attack?

L: Just when I see a pretty girl.

M: Anything else? Cancer? High blood pressure? Liver trouble or kidney trouble?

L: Well, in January 1944 I had a bad cold. They gave me sulfa, and by mistake the doctor gave me a dose four times as much as he should of. It burned up my kidneys. He told me I'd remember that forever. He's right. Sometimes I have a hard time passing my urine, and I remember that doctor and his sulfa.

M: Any other problems? Allergies?

L: Just to grass. I can't do that. But my good wife mows the lawn. She can hardly push the mower, but I don't get allergies then.

M: Good for her.

- What is this patient's chief complaint?
- What have his recent symptoms been?

Discussion

This doctor listens well. He uses facilitatory nods and hums and easily gets his patient talking about the problems at hand. Especially in the early portion of the interview this skill is invaluable. However, his patient tends to tell stories of medical care and of his own theories that, while edifying, still need symptomatic clarification. The doctor needs some device to help redirect his patient to current symptoms. The easiest is just to ask for what you want—current symptoms.

M: Mr. L, I need to understand better. Have you recently been having any symptoms other than the black stools and the dizziness and the sour pain in the pit of your stomach?

L: No, but back in 1944 I had . . .

M: No, wait a second, Mr. L. I need you to stick to NOW for a bit. Recently, any other symptoms at all? Pain? Shortness of breath? Cough? Nausea? Any others?

L: Well, the cough and breathing trouble of course. That's just the emphysema. I got that because of all that smoke in the trains.

M: Ah, that's right, you mentioned emphysema. Let's talk about the cough and the breathing trouble.

L: Well, in 1944, I started . . .

M: No, wait a bit. Mr. L, I need you to tell me first about what's happening now. Tell me about the cough and the breathing recently.

Thus, it is possible to direct the patient with a 50-year-old story to the present and to symptoms. Of course it is important to recognize that we are hearing a story important to this patient when he tells us his 1944 saga. He believes that illness is the root of his trouble. But we do need to hear current symptoms to get anywhere in our diagnostic and therapeutic efforts.

Case 39

NOT FIT FOR A HUMAN BEING

It was one of those days. Dr. X realized that he had been hating his work all day long. He hated dealing with the patients who were sick and hated those who were well. He hated the people he didn't like very much and hated having to talk to the people he always loved to see. His entire day in the office had been a matter of striking names off his list and hoping to get through to the end of the day. Now, thinking he had only two more patients to see, he stopped to see the posted list in his office and discovered that his assistants had added three more penciled-in, late callers, all needing to be seen today.

He felt overwhelmed by despair. Even a cup of coffee and three gingersnaps did little to help. Feeling weighed down by duty, he went to see his next patient.

- Have you ever been in such a state?
- Is it a frequent frame of mind for you?
- Is Dr. X suffering burnout?
- What do you advise?

Discussion

I think that good doctors are perpetually in a state of burnout. They are using themselves up and sometimes come up empty. I first understood this after reading Michael Balint's *The Doctor, His Patient, and the Illness* [50]. He talks about treating the patient with surgery, with medicines, and with the person of the physician. At first I thought the third treatment modality was a metaphor, but now I think it is literal. You really treat your patients with your own substance, and sometimes there is little or none of it left. You may notice this state when you come home and have no humanity left for your spouse or your children. Or, like Dr. X in this story, you may notice it during your workday. Is this a call for psychotherapy or for a vacation? Probably both would be a good idea, but it seems to go with the territory. What to do? Dr. X told his patients.

X: Hello, Mr. A. How are you?
A: Pretty good, Doc. How are you doing?
X: Well, actually, this is not a good day for me. I am pretty much of a bear, and I should not be allowed to talk to human beings. I'm not fit for a human being. In fact, I probably should be sent to my room. I expect I will be OK in another day or so, but today I will have to give you short shrift.
A: That's OK, Doc. You usually spend time with me. I can stand it today.

Does that sound outlandish to you? If so, what is so remarkable? The doctor being in an untherapeutic mood? The doctor explaining it to his patient? His patient being so tolerant? We are often in nontherapeutic states, and if so, we do a lot better telling our patients than confusing them by our actions. I find that my patients will forgive a great deal. It might be a different matter if we were a mess every day, but once in a while even doctors get to be dysfunctional.

Martin Lipp has written about doctors, patients, and failed expectations in *The Bitter Pill* [51]. He says that our work is really rough and that we have good reason to have bad days. He says,

"When we can, we must try to let our patients help us, by letting them know how hard we are struggling and with which forces." I do not believe that it is our patients' job to heal our wounds, but that it is acceptable to have wounds and occasionally to let on that we are not impervious or omnipotent.

Case 40

WHAT DID DR. REYNOLDS THINK

Mrs. Q has persistent nonspecific abdominal pain but two years ago surprised her doctors by hemorrhaging from a large gastric ulcer. Her pain now seems hard to define, and she has no abnormal laboratory results or physical findings. An upper GI x-ray series shows only the deformity of a past partial gastrectomy. Accordingly she has been sent to see a gastroenterologist, Dr. Reynolds, who was to perform an endoscopic examination. She then returned to her primary care doctor, Dr. X.

Dr. X: Hello, Mrs. Q. How have you been?

Q: Just about the same, doctor. The pain is just the same.

X: Un huh. And did Dr. Reynolds do the endoscopy?

Q: Oh yes. He did that two weeks ago. He said he'd talk to you. He said I ought to come back in three months for a colonoscopy. What did he think? What did Dr. Reynolds tell you? What did Dr. Reynolds think?

X: Hmm. I don't think he called me. Let me look through your chart to see if he wrote a letter. . . . . No, I don't find anything. I guess we've had a communication gap. I will call him.

Q: That's strange. It was two weeks ago.

X: Yes. Well, hmm. So it was. Hmm.

- What is Dr. X thinking?
- How can we prevent these complications?

Discussion

Dr. X says his initial response was anger with Dr. Reynolds for leaving him in the lurch this way. He then did call Dr. Reynolds and learned that a consultation letter had been dictated, perhaps not yet mailed. Dr. R was a little annoyed that he was being questioned on the phone about the material he had so clearly laid out in his letter. Dr. X was miffed that he had not been informed prior to the patient's visit to his office. He suggested to Dr. R that a phone call would have been more helpful and asked that he be called in the future as soon as an evaluation was completed. Dr. X thought Dr. R was less helpful than he should be as a consultant, and Dr. R thought that Dr. X should have told him what he wanted before sending the patient to him. Neither was very happy with the other.

Those of us who ask for consultative help from our colleagues and those of us who give such help probably need to spend more time thinking about the connection we make with each other. The consultee should clarify his desires and needs, and the consultant needs to consider the use that his help will be put to. I think there is no good replacement for face-to-face or at least telephone conversation, but I believe request forms can be devised and used that could help clarify our desires and needs to the consultant. Do we want the consultant to take over care of the patient? Do we want therapy to be withheld until we discuss the matter together? Do we want a phone call right away? We need to specify what we want.

Now that you've experienced this failure of doctor-to-doctor communication, you must remember that you still have a patient to talk with. It's fine to let your patient know that you understand how exasperating such a turn of events is to her. Then it is OK to admit your own exasperation too. Just avoid casting too much blame. If you do point out Dr. Reynold's faults to your patient, you will probably later find the miscommunication to have been mostly your own fault and will have to eat your words. It always seems to go that way with me. So my advice is to stick with what's happening now and try to solve the patient's problems. Then later you can chat with Dr. Reynolds and try to fix the communication process so that it doesn't go wrong in just this exact fashion again.

Case 41

AN INTERESTING CASE

Dr. Z's wife was ill. She suffered from a genetic disorder, acute intermittent porphyria. Now she was ill with nausea, abdominal and back pain, and great weakness. She had taken in very little fluid for several days and seemed to be getting weaker and weaker.

Dr. Z brought Mrs. Z to the emergency room, where she was to be examined by the emergency doctor, Dr. A.

A: Hi, Z. How are you?
Z: Not so hot. My wife's sick.
A: Oh! What's up?
Z: She's getting dehydrated, I think. She has porphyria. Acute intermittent porphyria.
A: Oh, how interesting. That must be very interesting for you.
Z: No, mostly it's just scary. I'm worried about her.
A: Still, that's a pretty rare disorder. I can imagine how interesting it is.

- Have you ever BEEN an interesting case?
- Has someone you loved BEEN an interesting case?
- What might Dr. A do for Dr. Z that would be therapeutic?

Discussion

I think that what Dr. Z most wants from Dr. A is careful attention to Mrs. Z. Nothing else will do. But in the process Dr. A could try a tiny dose of empathy. He might ask himself how Dr. Z is feeling and probably could come up with an empathic remark like: "Gosh, I can imagine. You must be quite concerned." And then: "Let me go talk to her right away."

But the concept of an "interesting patient" is pretty interesting itself. What in the world do we mean by it? I think it usually is employed to refer to a rare disorder or to a real puzzle that we haven't the foggiest notion how to approach or to a patient whom we have no hope of helping. Often the "interesting" appellation is triggered by the rarity of the disorder. And why is that so interesting to us? Or to reverse the puzzle, why are we not interested in common disorders?

Twenty-five years ago, as a resident on the neurology service, my attending was Dr. Ed Lewin. I remember telling him about a boy who had hyperuricemia and chewed off his fingers. There was even a name for the syndrome. "This is really interesting," I said. "No it isn't," Ed replied. "You'll never see another similar case. Don't you have a case of a seizure disorder or a fainter or someone with a stroke? Now THAT would be interesting." I think he was right. We have to find interest in our daily work or we go crazy, and our patients suffer.

Then there is the strange perversion of medical education that leads doctors to assume that their patients have an obligation to interest the doctor. I've heard patients apologize for not bringing a "more interesting problem" to the doctor. And surely, in my teaching hospital it is commonplace for the house staff to sign off the care of a patient when little is happening and the patient is "no longer of teaching interest." They then can avoid having to deal with the chronic problems that cause practitioners of medicine to lose sleep and hair. I've even heard young doctors commenting on patients with AIDS and weird infectious complications, saying that they had seen several similar patients and this one was no longer "interesting." Wow! The biggest and worst epidemic since the fourteenth century is not interesting!

So here are my conclusions: First, it is not the obligation of any patient to interest his doctor. The patient has come for help, not to provide entertainment. Second, rare is not synonymous with interesting. It behooves us to find great interest in the most common problems. Third, no one wants to be sick, neither with rare diseases, nor with common ones, and none of us wants our loved ones to be sick.

It is true that patients who have unusual disorders attract more attention in many medical centers [52, 53]. That's not altogether a good thing, since they may then also have more complications from more tests and studies. But if the patient gets pleasure out of being a focus of attention, having a rare disease might be the ticket. Otherwise, forget it.

Is this a bit too preachy? Could be, since I was Dr. Z and didn't find it at all comforting for my wife to be "an interesting case."

Case 42

SPEAK UP!

The physician was a kind, gentle person who spoke very softly. He was attending to an elderly patient in the hospital.

Dr. X: Have you had any pain in your legs?
Mr. B: No, I don't think so.
X: We are concerned because you had that arterial obstruction in your right leg.
B: Uh huh.
X: So we think we ought to redo the noninvasive studies.
B: Uh huh.
X: Is that what you think?
B: Uh huh.

Another physician in the room, knowing that the patient had a hearing problem, interrupted.

Dr. Y: Mr. B, did you hear what Dr. X just said?
B: Well, not exactly, no. I heard some of it.
Y: I think you have to speak more loudly to Mr. B. He is a little hard of hearing.
X: [Every bit as softly] I was just asking about your legs. Are they bothering you?
B: [Looking up attentively] Uh.

When asked why he spoke so softly to a patient who was elderly and hearing-impaired, Dr. X said that it was his mother's fault.

X: My mother always told me to be respectful of older people. And that includes not shouting at the person you respect.

- What about that? Is it acceptable to speak loudly to an older person? Would it be disrespectful? What would the patient think?

Discussion

There is no communication rule that shouldn't be broken if it is interfering with good communication. We must consider our goals and not stumble over any rigid rule of how we get there. Surely it is important to raise our voices when a person is hearing-impaired.

In fact, when elderly patients are asked what doctors should do differently, the first request is "Speak up!" Many patients are shy about admitting difficulty in hearing, even if it costs them an understanding of what the doctor is saying. Sometimes they count on a relative being present and remembering what the doctor said.

We can ask our patients to tell us what they understood of what we said. If we do that, we will often be surprised at how little they heard and how little they understand. The problem isn't just hearing. It does little good to explain if we are unheard or misunderstood. We have to check out our results here as elsewhere.

Case 43

THE TREACHEROUS K-Y JELLY DISASTER

Dr. X, a senior medical resident, was examining a new patient in the hospital. During the history and physical examination, his supervisor, the medical program director, had been seated in a corner of the room, taking this opportunity to observe his resident's clinical skills.

The physical examination was nearly complete. Dr. X removed an ancient tube of lubricant from his medical bag and absentmindedly tidied up the tube, squeezing it from the bottom, as he explained the next task to the patient.

X: What I'm going to do is a rectal examination. I will have you roll on your side, and I will insert a gloved finger in . . .

At that moment the bottom of the tube popped open and the lubricant flowed out, running down the doctor's white-coated arm.

The medical director began to laugh. The patient gaped at this spectacle, and then he too began to laugh. The resident turned to stone.

X: I uh. I uh, that is . . . hmm.
Patient: You better mop that up with some paper towels, Doc.
X: Yes. Well, uh, hmm. [After staring at his arm for 30 seconds] I uh, I guess we will have to stop now. I'll clean this all up, and I'll come back later to do the rectal exam.

Twelve years later, this ex-resident remembers the event with mixed feelings, but mostly humor. "If I only could have laughed then," he says, "I might have been much better off."

• What do you think? What do you do when you have stumbled over your own feet and your patient is laughing at you?

Discussion

Most physicians, even the most egalitarian, seem to function best with some distance between them and their patients. We may not feel comfortable with the godlike posture that some of our predecessors maintained, but we may need a certain professional distance from the patient to feel most comfortable in our role. That distance is abridged dramatically when we get caught in an awkward situation.

For this physician in training who was confident of his skills but still uneasy with being observed by the big boss, an accident of this sort was humiliating and devastating.

Judith Martin, a.k.a. "Miss Manners," talks about "Acts of God," events that are so embarrassing that good manners require the observer to disregard their occurrence. Too bad that neither the program director nor the patient understood this principle of etiquette. I was that program director in 1980 and have to make a belated apology to this physician for my guffaws. I wish I had been more empathetic with the resident in our postexercise discussion. I'm not sure now just what I said to him in 1980, but I suspect that I was still savoring and he was still agonizing over the happening. On the other hand, we both now realize that such an event is a miraculous opportunity to acknowledge our humanity by sharing a good laugh at ourselves.

I recall catching my thumb between the footrest and the bed of a patient I was examining. Wow! Did that hurt! I quickly expressed my distress with several short Anglo-Saxon words. My patient remained calm and accepting. "That's exactly what I say when I do that, Doc," he said.

Case 44

A RATTLESNAKE BIT ME ON THE KNEE

Dr. I: Mr. S, how old are you?

S: Eighty-three.

I: And how have you been doing all those 83 years?

S: I've done a lot of things.

I: That's good. How did you land here in the hospital?

S: I was hurting. It hurt in my chest, and it got into my left arm.

I: Ever before?

S: Well I was hospitalized in WXY once for five days. I went in one day, and they said I had a bad heart attack. But I didn't see a doctor until Saturday five days later when he came and stood in the doorway and said to me, "You're always running up to Mayo's, so why don't you get up there now."

I: So you had a heart attack then.

S: Well I don't really know. My son-in-law brought me here, and Dr. Q says I never had a heart attack.

I: OK. How often do you have pain?

S: I had a hiatal hernia once. They diagnosed it at the Mayo Clinic. I don't have pain but maybe once a year.

I: Do you use nitroglycerin?

S: I used three on Sunday.

I: Then you had that pain. Tell me, on a scale of one to ten, how bad was the pain?

S: That's like rating altitudes. It depends on where you're standing.

I: OK. Did you have shortness of breath? Can you sleep flat? Do you get leg swelling? Edema?

S: Sometimes I swell a little, my legs . . .

I: Palpitations?

S: My heart started skipping beats when I was about 17. It does that occasionally. Once my heart slowed down to about 42, they said.

I: Did you pass out?

S: Just once 40 years ago.

I: What do you do?

S: Mostly just play cards. Then I was going to tell you that my knee hasn't been right since a rattlesnake bit it.

I: Your knee isn't right?

S: Yeah, I was about to have knee surgery back in May when something hit me.

I: What?

S: My lungs filled up.

I: Really? Did you have pneumonia? Heart failure?

S: I don't know, but they put off the knee operation.

I: Any allergies?

S: Just penicillin. It gives me a rash.

I: So the chest pain brought you in.

S: It's really the knee that gives me the most trouble. It hurts and won't work.

- What is the theme of this interview?
- If this were a dance, what would you advise the choreographer?

Discussion

It is hard to analyze an interview that is as chaotic as this. There seems to be no clear theme and no clear direction that the process is taking. It is even hard to understand where the chaos comes from, with the doctor usually blaming the patient, perhaps calling him a "poor historian."

My theory is that this sort of zigzag interview is largely the result of the doctor's process. This doctor, for example, specializes in questions and asks them in rapid-fire order. The patient never gets much time to tell his story, to complete his thoughts, or even to finish a sentence. If you go back to the doctor's opening, "How did you land here in the hospital?" you will see that the doctor's next question came about five seconds later: "Ever before?" That second question is a sensible one and needs an eventual answer, but need not be asked so fast. One of the results of this haste is that the doctor takes the patient's first utterance as the chief complaint. It may not be! Robert Burack and Robert Carpenter [54] showed that the first complaint is often not the chief complaint. Even if this were the reason he came to the hospital, his most bothersome symptom (the technical definition of a "chief complaint") may only surface later. In fact, this patient's chief complaint is really his knee pain.

Haste seems to me to be the primary cause of much of this interview's flaws. Consider the wonderful opportunity for empathy that was missed when the patient told how he had been abandoned in a hospital in WXY. Imagine how he must have felt to be spoken to by the doctor in the manner he describes! Imagine how he feels right now, remembering that treatment! The doctor misses the opportunity to respond to the first with "That must have felt awful!" and to the second with "I can imagine you are still angry about it." This doctor is smart and alert; her rushing causes her to miss an opportunity.

What of her response to "My lungs filled up"? Instead of asking for the symptoms of that event, she asks for diagnoses: "Pneumonia? Heart failure?" Again, I suspect that haste leads to that error of focus. We all know that we need to hear symptoms more than diagnoses.

Choreographically, we need to slow this boogie to a waltz. Then the two partners need to get in step.

Case 45

TOMORROW

Mr. N, a 74-year-old man, came to the office complaining of two weeks of dreadful pain in his left thigh and knee. Sometimes the pain radiated into his lower back, but most of the time he felt it in his knee, especially when he tried to walk. The rest of his history was unrelated to the current event, and he denied any unusual activity or trauma. Many years before he had a lumbar laminectomy for disc disease. The physical examination showed a definite limp and a marked decrease in his usual mobility, some limitation of movement at the left knee and the left hip, but nothing else of note. He was sent for x-rays of the lumbar spine, left hip, and left knee. He then returned home to use heat and analgesics and to await a phone call from his doctor about the radiographs. The next day his doctor called.

Dr. X: Nick? This is Dr. X. I'm calling to tell you about your x-rays.

N: Oh? How were they, Doctor?

X: Not too bad actually. There is some arthritis in all these areas but no broken hip or other terrible problem. I think we have to keep doing what we're doing now. How has the pain been?

N: Some better and some worse. It'll be OK for a while and then gets worse again.

X: Ah.

N: And you know I'm trying to sell my house. They say that I'll lose my homeowner's insurance when I sell my house.

X: And?

N: And I'm pretty mad about it. I'm really steaming!

X: And the relationship to your leg pain is?

N: No relationship. It's just that's what I'm concerned about. I'm living with my daughter now.

X: Nick, do you know who I am?

N: Of course I know. You're my doctor.

X: OK, I was wondering if you thought I was your realtor or your insurance man.

N: No, I know who's who. I'm not losing my mind, just my homeowner's insurance.

X: OK. How about continuing your medicines for the leg and calling me in a few days?

N: OK. That sounds all right.

- How's this for an example of doctors hearing their patients?
- What next?
- Why "Tomorrow"?

Discussion

Why "Tomorrow"? Because there usually is a tomorrow, and that's a good time to do what we failed to do today.

Dr. X shunted his patient's concerns altogether off the medical main line. I agree that they were probably not medical. But we can't disregard our patients' stories lightly. If we do, we risk missing important information and we risk alienating our patients. If we can't listen to what they have to say, we discount their concerns and diminish their trust in us. We don't have to fix those concerns, just hear them.

Dr. X thought about this conversation overnight and realized that he had given his patient short shrift. So he called him the next day. Their conversation was brief:

X: Hello Nick, this is Dr. X. I was thinking about our conversation yesterday.

N: Oh, yeah. What about it?

X: Well, just that I thought I hadn't been very patient with your story about your house and the insurance. I realize that you are truly very concerned about that matter.

N: Yeah, well it isn't so bad maybe. Today I heard that I get a three-month overlap. So if I can sell the place within three months I'm OK.

X: I see. Then maybe it isn't so bad for you.

N: No, Doc. I'm OK. Thanks for calling.

X: You're welcome.

How does that sound? Nothing really accomplished? Maybe, but I think apologizing for our errors is terribly important and that it does wonders for future interactions. I haven't presented a controlled trial of apology here, and one case can't be its own control. Still I bet we could tell the value of appropriate apologies in a well-controlled prospective study if we could get one funded.

Case 46

WHO ARE YOU ANYWAY?

A new patient enters the office suite and stands in front of the reception counter. Behind the counter are seated two staff people. One is turned away, checking names on a schedule book. The other, facing the patient, is talking on the telephone. There is no signal from either that they have noticed the new person. The new person stands still for three minutes. Finally the telephoner finishes her conversation and, without looking at him, hands him a form.

Staff Person: Fill this out.

New Person: Can I have a pen?

SP: [Silently places a ballpoint pen on the counter.]

NP: [Handing over the form] Is this all right?

SP: Have a seat. Dr. X will see you in a few minutes.

- OK, this brief interchange doesn't really fit in "The Doctor Did It," does it? But what about "The Doctor's Staff Did It"? That's close enough for me.
- What message does this patient get?
- How could we do it better?

Discussion

James Thurber, in an essay on grammar, said that he thought it was impolite to address someone you have known for many years by "Whom are you anyway?" That line has always seemed the epitome of silliness to me, and I treasure it. But I am afraid that we often treat our patients just as impolitely at the first opportunity they have to meet us.

The engagement process is critical to medical communication, and it begins before the patient meets his new doctor. In fact, our telephone answerers, appointment schedulers, and office receptionists reflect the quality of care that we offer.

This doctor's front office staff act as if they had been trained to discount and discourage prospective patients. Their message to the patient seems to be "You are not important to us. We don't care who you are and can hardly be bothered to speak with you."

What would work better?

One receptionist whose work I admire pays attention to the daily schedule and knows whom she is expecting. Her dialogue with a new patient, accompanied by a direct look and a vigorous display of personality, goes like this:

K: Are you John Jones?
NP: Yes, I am.
K: Oh good! That's just who you are supposed to be! I'm Katie. I need you to fill out this form.

In that short interchange, she has told the patient that she is glad to see him, was looking forward to his appearance, and has a little humor to spare. He knows that he is known, even by his name, and begins to form a relationship with her. And she still gets the paperwork done!

Physicians often note that they have patients who are polite to them but who seem to abuse their staff. I have surmised that such a patient has real grievances against the physician but feels it is too dangerous to blame the doctor. Maybe not. Perhaps the patient is angry with the staff because the staff mistreat him. If they disregard, discount, or discourage the patient, I can understand his being unhappy and even angry.

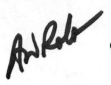

Case 47

THAT JUST HAPPENS SOMETIMES

The patient is a 50-year-old medical journalist who fell on the ice, injuring her right wrist. Her wrist was quite tender and painful, but worse, she suffered chills and weakness during the next 24 hours before consulting an orthopedist. The surgeon examined her wrist, obtained an x-ray, and splinted the injury. "Nothing to worry about," he said. "No fracture. You'll be fine in a few days. Come back to see me in two weeks."

As he predicted, the wrist was pain-free within three days, and the patient removed her splint. Not convinced that she needed any more medical attention, she still returned in two weeks because she had been so puzzled about the plethora of symptoms she had suffered at the time of her initial injury.

Ms. A: Hello, Dr. X. My wrist seems fine. As you predicted, it was pain-free in three days, and I took off the splint.

Dr. X: [Examining the wrist] Great! I don't think I have to see you until your next disaster.

A: Well, what I'm really concerned about is the chills I had. When I fell and injured my wrist, I had chills for 24 hours, shaking chills, and I felt generally miserable, weak, faint, altogether not myself.

X: Yes. Well, the arm seems to have healed up just fine.

A: And what caused the other symptoms?

X: That just happens sometimes.

A: But I still don't see . . .

X: Nothing to worry about. It just happens. Bye now.

Ms. A was not satisfied with the answer but felt ambivalent about going on. She no longer felt sick and did agree that her wrist had healed. She thought that her doctor had cared for her wrist in an appropriate manner, yet his answer to her concerns seemed inadequate. Paradoxically, she left his office feeling worse.

- What's going on?
- What could Dr. X do?

Discussion

What's the doctor's problem? Can't say, "I don't know"? Doesn't want to "waste time on the patient's concerns"? Doesn't understand that the least serious illnesses and symptoms may require the most discussion and education? It could be any of these. But clearly the patient feels discounted by the doctor's abruptness.

Let's consider these alternative actions. First, however, it seems necessary that Dr. X stop and consider his own feelings. He could have an internal dialogue, perhaps something like this:

X1: What's the trouble, X?

X2: I don't know. This woman doesn't seem satisfied with a perfectly good result.

X1: And how are you feeling?

X2: Not very appreciated. And rushed. And uncertain. I don't know how to satisfy her.

X1: Mmm. Tough situation! What about letting her know that you can hear her concerns.

X2: How would I do that?

X1: How about just saying, "I can hear your concerns. You're feeling fine now but are concerned about how sick you felt at the time of the injury."

X2: Oh! OK.

X: Ms. A, I can hear your concern. You're feeling fine now, but you are concerned about how sick you felt at the time of your injury.

A: That's it, doctor. I felt weak and had those terrible chills. I thought chilling was a symptom of infection, not a sprained wrist. It frightened me. I wondered if there was something else wrong we hadn't recognized.

X: I see. And those symptoms—have they bothered you recently?

A: No, Doctor, just for the first 24 hours, two weeks ago.

X2: Now what? I think she sounds less antagonistic now, but what do I do now? I don't know why she had chills. I haven't the foggiest idea!

X1: How about telling her that?

X2: Oh! OK.

X: Well, Ms. A, in truth I don't know why you had chills. I have heard that story before with fairly simple injuries, but I don't know the explanation.

A: I see. Well, that's reassuring. Do you think I had some sort of an infection?

X: Probably not. Anyway, I think we ought not do anything more unless the symptoms recur. OK?

A: Sure. That sounds right to me. Thank you, Doctor.

X: Don't mention it. It was a pleasure.

What are the take-home lessons?

First, when you are troubled by an interaction, stop and consider your own feelings first. Then, try to understand where the patient is coming from. What are the patient's feelings and concerns?

Next, try to let your patient know that you have heard and understood those concerns. It usually pays to rename them so that the patient understands the level of your understanding. You may need help to further understand her concerns; is there any specific fear that she wants to be assured about? You have to ask to find out.

Third, it is reasonable to admit ignorance, much better than some sort of cover-up statement like "That just happens sometimes." Even if you are, in the end, to say just that, an admission of ignorance comes first.

Finally, the least serious disorders do require the most explanation. This orthopedist probably can get by with a very brief explanation when the problem is a fractured femur. He should try to explain a viral upper respiratory infection that briefly. Disaster! Part of the difficulty lies in the need to consider a human being rather than a bone. And part consists of the greater uncertainty inherent in human concerns.

Case 48

I HOPE I ANSWERED YOUR QUESTIONS ALL RIGHT

The resident physician was being observed as he performed a timed exercise, a history and physical examination that were expected to take 45 minutes. The faculty preceptor and the resident reviewed their expectations ahead of time and agreed that the event could not be comprehensive because of its time constraint. The resident was to allocate his time as he saw fit.

During the interview portion of the exercise, the resident paid exquisite attention to his patient. He listened attentively and offered good summations of the story at appropriate moments. He responded empathically to the emotional content, for example:

Patient A: I've been so weak that my wife has had to do everything for me. I'm not normally like that. I've always been strong and capable.
Dr. X: That must be hard on you to be so dependent.
A: Yes. It's hard to watch my wife do all the work.
X: I can imagine.

Because the history was complex, Dr. X allocated most of his time to it. He was left with less time than he wished for the physical examination and had to abridge his planned thorough evaluation. Even so, he ran over five minutes. Finally he began to close.

X: We're going to stop here.
A: OK.
X: I enjoyed talking to you.
A: Thanks. I enjoyed meeting you too. I'm still alive, I guess.
X: You are! I hope you get some of your activity level back [packing up his examination tools].
A: I hope I answered your questions all right.
X: Well, we're a little bit short on time.
A: Oh [discouraged and sad sounding]. OK.
X: Goodbye.
A: Goodbye.

• What happened at the very end?
• If you consider one of the initial interview tasks to be ENGAGEMENT with the patient, how does that relate to the tasks of ENDING the interview?

- Escaping from the patient's room at the end of an interchange seems problematic to many physicians. How does one best part with the patient?

Discussion

One way to consider this case is to examine the ending ceremony. Do you have such a ceremony? Is it one you have considered and can define? Whether you have or not, there is a need to bring the interaction to an end and to finish with both patient and doctor feeling good about the experience. It helps to think about the components of termination. I like to think of the exiting process as one similar to the engagement process at the beginning of the interview. When you start, do you introduce yourself to the patient? Use his name? Shake hands? Say what is to come next? You can and should do all those again at the end of your interaction.

Dr. X: Well, it's time to close up now. We're going to go as soon as I pack up my equipment.
A: OK.
X: It has been a real pleasure to meet you, Mr. A [offering his hand to shake with the patient].
A: I enjoyed talking with you too, Doctor.
X: I want to make sure that I left my name with you clearly. I'm Dr. X.
A: Yes, I remembered.
X: OK. Well, I'll be leaving. Is there anything you need before I go? Anything I can do to make you more comfortable?
A: No, I'm fine, Doctor.
X: Well then, goodbye for now.
A: Goodbye. Thank you, Doctor.

Then we have to consider the last little interchange of this original dialogue:

A: I hope I've answered your questions all right.
X: Well, we're a little short of time.

A more apt response by the physician might be:

X: You did just fine, Mr. A. Just fine.

How did this attentive physician miss his patient's request for reassurance? I suspect that the doctor had ceased to think about the patient and was focusing on his own needs and his own wishes to perform well. He was probably saying to himself, "I did pretty well, but I ran out of time and couldn't do all I had wished." So he answered Mr. A out of his own needs.

How might Dr. X prevent this sort of slip? I think there are at least two approaches. One is to learn an exit ceremony such as I've detailed. Or at least recognize that there is such a ceremony and that finishing an event has specific requirements. But for this physician whose strength is his focused attention to his patient, I think the remedy is just to continue that attention until the event is entirely over. The old pilot adage applies here: "The landing isn't over until the airplane is tied down." This airplane wasn't yet securely tied down.

7

Patience, Humility, and Compassion

patience *forbearance under stress, provocation, or indignity; toleration or magnanimity for the faults and affronts of others.*

humility *freedom from pride or arrogance. "We all need humility in the face of what we do not understand."*

compassion *a deep feeling for misery or suffering and the concomitant desire to promote its alleviation. Spiritual consciousness of the personal tragedy of another and selfless tenderness directed toward it.*

Webster's Third New International Dictionary,
Unabridged 1971

There is always room for more. Whatever skills we master, we will always need more. In the end, what we need most are the hardest skills to teach, skills so essential as to resemble personality features.

Find a medical text for me, please, that has a chapter on patience. Or a good controlled clinical trial of patience. But what do we need more of as physicians? From this word and this concept comes the root of the word we use for our clients, *patients*. What would you rather master, the prostaglandin sequence or patience? Which do your patients hope more to find in you? Which do you think is more often a critical lack?

The Greeks spoke about hubris, a state of pride. And pride was viewed by medieval Christian philosophers as the greatest of all the mortal sins. Who can have enough humility? Yet *hubris* is almost a defining character flaw for doctors, perhaps our chief occupational hazard.

And then, compassion. More than empathy, compassion allows the extra step we can go for a fellow human being. Twenty years ago I worked in the Denver General Hospital Emergency Department. One evening three physician colleagues and I watched a man enter the department through its swinging doors 100 feet away from us. He staggered toward us, weaving and bobbing, using the wall as a support. Finally he leaned on the wall and slithered to the floor. "Drunk as an owl," said one of my colleagues. We all nodded. Then one of the doctors detached himself from our group, walked down the hall, and helped the man to his feet. I remember wondering at the time what had been the matter with me. What was wrong that I hadn't seen the need of a fellow human and acted with a bit of compassion, as my colleague had done? I still remember that event with chagrin.

Compassion may ask us to return to do a task we missed doing the first time.

Compassion may be found in an act as simple as bringing a morning cup of coffee to a patient or making a telephone call that you might leave to another.

From compassion comes evidence of caring, evidence that makes all the difference. It is seldom a matter of "going an extra mile"; rather, as in my emergency room experience, another 20 yards may do.

Case 49

HER CAROTID ARTERY IS KILLING HER

Dr. X is on call this weekend. At 11 P.M. he received a message from his answering service to call Ms. Wilma, who is Dr. P's patient.

X: Hello, this is Dr. X. Is Ms. Wilma there?
W: Yes, Doctor. I'm Wilma.
X: Well I'm on call for your doctor, Dr. P. Can I help you?
W: Actually, Dr. P isn't my doctor. He's Sharon's doctor.
X: Sharon?
W: Yes, I'm calling about her. Her carotid artery is killing her. I think maybe she ought to go to the hospital and be seen by a specialist.
X: Why is that?
W: Because it's killing her, that's why. It could rupture and cause a stroke.
X: I see. I didn't make myself clear, I guess. I meant why did you think it was her carotid artery?
W: Because I don't think it's anything else. Should I take her to the hospital?
X: Maybe. Perhaps I could talk to her first. Can you put her on the phone?
W: Oh, no, I can't. She isn't here. She was here earlier, but she went home.
X: So you are calling for her since you are concerned about her carotid artery, but she isn't there.
W: Yes.
X: Well, how about if you give me her number, and I'll call her.
W: OK. She might not be home yet though. She said she might stop off on the way.
X: Well, tell me her number anyway.
W: OK. It's . . . just let me look here a minute. [Pause] OK, it's 333-3333.
X: I'll call her.
W: Thank you, Doctor.

S: Hello? [Very noisy background.]
X: Hello, I'm Dr. X. Ms. Wilma suggested that I call you. I'm on call for Dr. P.
S: Yes, he's my doctor. WILL SOMEONE TURN THAT TV OFF?
X: I didn't get your last name, I'm sorry.
S: Sparks. I'm Sharon Sparks.

X: OK. What's up, Ms. Sparks?

S: Mostly my carotid artery, I guess. It's likely to blow my head off.

X: Can you tell me what symptoms you've . . .

S: Sometimes I think it will just explode. ROBERT, TURN THAT OFF!

X: Uh, could you tell me what symptoms . . .

S: Symptoms? You mean like how it hurts?

X: Yeah.

S: It hurts a lot, that's what. My whole head pounds, and I'm sick as a dog. I couldn't keep anything down for dinner.

X: So we're talking about headache then.

S: Yeah. I used to get these every week, but since Dr. P put me on propranol, I haven't. Then I ran out last month, and this one has been a humdoozie.

X: OK, I'm beginning to get the picture.

Discussion

I think that Dr. X did really well, much better than I usually do in like circumstances.

I'm usually asleep when these calls come, and having just fallen asleep, I am at my worst when awakened. To find that I have to deal with a sequence of my least favorite problems provides a real test for my patience. In this sequence:

1. Another person calls for the patient, a person who doesn't know the symptoms well.

2. The patient is at another location, requiring at least one more phone call.

3. The friend assumes that I don't have adequate skills to handle the problem, that her friend needs "to see a specialist."

4. The patient is in a noisy environment, and neither she nor I can concentrate with the high level of background interference.

5. The patient (and her friend before her) want to tell me her diagnosis rather than her symptoms.

Confronted with this, my greatest task is to remain patient. It does not help if I lose my patience and express my annoyance with either of these two people. I might, later on, have to explain that I can't sort the matter out over the phone or at that time and make arrangements to see the patient tomorrow, but it is no use to get angry at their misunderstanding my role and my needs.

Patience seems to be my greatest need as I practice medicine, and it is the skill I had the least training in at home or at school. Surely doctors get into trouble more from lack of patience than from inability to reproduce the complement cascade from memory. Why aren't we tested on patience/impatience? I will put patience in the category of great themes that are critical for the practice of medicine but are seldom mentioned, like the fact that we are going to work with sick people, people who are suffering from loss and fear and increasing disability. Nobody ever told me about that. My teachers assumed the daily practice of medicine was like childbirth: The uninitiated have no context for apprehending the truth of the experience, and those who do it find it too profound to describe.

Case 50

I JUST DON'T WANT TO KNOW

S: I'm feeling really fine, Fred. I have my usual hay fever, but otherwise I'm fine. I've been very active, gardening, working on the foundation, just fine.

F: OK, Stan. What sort of poisons are you putting into your body?

S: You mean the alcohol? I still drink about three cocktails a day, but they are dilute. I don't put a shot of whiskey in each.

F: And more some days?

S: Just when we go out. Josh and I go out maybe once a week, and I might have another one or two drinks those nights.

F: Remind me of your relationship with Josh.

S: We're just good friends. He's my best friend. We were lovers once but not now. Josh just found out that he's HIV positive. That's been a shock. He's feeling fine though. They started him on AZT.

F: Let's see. You're 63 now.

S: Josh is just 48. His family knows that he's gay, but they don't believe it.

F: Don't believe it?

S: Yeah. "Maybe the right woman will come along one day."

F: I see. So he's positive for HIV.

S: He has been a lot more active sexually than I have.

F: We've never tested you for HIV.

S: Yes. I really don't want to be tested. I don't want to know.

F: We can do some good things if we know. And you might be negative, you know.

S: That's what I think. I've never had much exposure. I've been nearly celibate, and I only did anal sex about twice ever.

F: When were you and Josh lovers?

S: Oh that was more than two years ago. We're just friends now. Sometimes we go on trips together.

F: So you probably were lovers when he was infected. And I see that you have lost about ten pounds since last year.

S: That's probably because I don't eat any fats any more. I eat almost a purely vegetarian diet now.

F: OK, let's go on and do a good examination, and then we can talk about the blood test.

[A complete examination reveals no abnormalities but the weight loss.]

S: Have you heard about that new blood test to look for early prostate cancer?

F: Yes, that's the PSA, prostate-specific antigen. We do that. And I would include it in a routine blood survey right now for you, but the more important test to do is the HIV antibody. We really ought to know if you are positive, and if that were true, we'd want to monitor your T_4 cell count. At a certain point it makes a lot of sense to start on AZT and even on *Pneumocystis* prophylaxis. Stan, that's really what I think we ought to do.

S: I know all that. I am surrounded by people with AIDS and

HIV infection. I really can't stand finding out about me now. I have to be the strong person for all these others, for Josh. I wouldn't have anyone to be there for me.

F: Nobody? No other friends?

S: Oh yeah, there are some. But I always feel better being the strong person. I always have been that way.

F: What would you say if you were in my shoes? Is there anything I can say that will help you?

S: I'd probably say the same things you are saying.

F: I would like you to know that I'm planning on being here for you. I won't desert you whatever you decide to do and whatever happens. I care about you and I'm fond of you.

S: I know that Fred. I just don't think I can do it right now.

F: Would you think about it for a week or so and come back to talk with me?

S: OK, I'll do that. Maybe I'll talk to the psychologist I consulted in the past. He was helpful.

F: OK.

S: I'll think about it. But I think that I can't do the test now. I just don't want to know.

- What leads patients to follow the doctor's advice when their initial impulse is to avoid that recommendation?
- What would you do to help convince Stan?
- By the way, is your office known as "AIDS friendly"?

Discussion

I suppose the name for this phenomenon is denial. What we don't know won't hurt us. If we don't name it, we don't really have it.

This man is an old friend of mine. I knew him 20 years ago, before he began to see me as his physician. He played with my children when they were small. I am very fond of him, and I find it hard to think of him having AIDS. I want to deny the possibility, much as he does.

How frightened and vulnerable Stan must feel right now. How hard to expose himself to one more threat, the threat of certain knowledge. How hard for the doctor who wants to help and shares Stan's urge to deny the possibility of this life-threatening disease.

What to do to help the patient accept the best therapy and best medical approach? Do we really know that approach? How to convince him? If, as it seems, he is already convinced intellectually, how can we allay his anxieties?

What will happen in one week? Will anything change?

The most powerful force that has been discovered in doctor-patient relationships is the patient's perception of the doctor's degree of concern. That perception is the most effective change agent we have. We must identify and name the painful areas, offer help, and evince our real concern. These days, when everyone in every walk of life is talking about "care," when used car dealers, shoe salesmen, and graphic designers join with fast food chains and nursing home administrations in claiming to "care about" their clients, the term may seem hackneyed and clichéd. But the concept is still the vital force for therapeutic change.

By the way, as I thought of our visit, I wished that I had given Stan a hug. I think maybe he could have used a little bit of a hug. He isn't one for effusive gestures, and I would have had just to drape one arm loosely over his shoulders, nothing more. I don't think I avoided a hug because I am threatened by Stan's sexuality; I just didn't think of it. Maybe next time. Because, as I think of it, I realize that Stan, for all his usual moral strength and fortitude, was sad and grieving and needed whatever support I could give him, including a hug.

Two weeks later Stan returned, agreed to the blood test, and we were both cheered to find it was negative. I asked him what made him decide to get the test, and do you know what he said? He said that it was my evident concern for him that did the trick.

Case 51

WILL HE GET BETTER?

John is a 13-year-old boy who, riding without a seat belt, suffered a severe closed head injury in an automobile crash. He sustained several fractures that have nearly healed now, about three months after his accident, but he still is at a very low cognitive level. He lies in bed, seeming awake, with wandering divergent eyes that do not focus on anyone or anything. He is mute but for moans and groans. He does not respond to anyone with any evidence of recognition. He breathes regularly, and his tracheostomy has been allowed to close. He is fed through a gastrostomy tube.

His mother is a frequent visitor at the bedside and often confronts nursing and medical staff about his prognosis. They note that nothing they tell her seems to satisfy her and that she asks the same questions over and over.

Mrs. R: How is John doing?
Nurse Patience: Not too bad. You know his fevers have been down now for several days.
R: Will he get better? Is he going to be all right? Will he get better?
P: Well, we never want to give up hope. And we're working with him in therapy. But it's been three months now, and we don't expect a lot of improvement.
R: I don't understand. They said that he'd get better here when they transferred him from St. Otherplace. They said you'd be able to help. Is he going to get well?
P: Well, he might do a little better. We hope he will eventually be able to sit up in a chair without falling.
R: But will he get well?

• This isn't the first request for information Mrs. R has made. What keeps her from understanding her son's bad prognosis? What should we do?

Discussion

I believe this problem may be so awful that no solution will serve.

Mrs. R may be confused. As a parent I can understand wanting to be misled. She may be the victim of misleading overhopeful prior communications. First of all, the accident was then more recent and the future prognosis less clear. Second, on transfer out of the acute care hospital to our rehabilitation facility, the staff didn't want to have to argue with their patient's family about a transfer to a lesser facility so they may have painted the rehabilitation hospital a rosy hue, extolling its facilities, its staff, and its benefits. Finally, the staff at the rehabilitation hospital themselves need exaggerated hope to do their work with so many patients in such bad straits. On admission they may have led John's mother to expect a miracle. None was forthcoming.

Nevertheless, I don't think Mrs. R needs or will benefit much from any more explanation. It will continue to fall upon deaf ears. She can't hear the bad news. She will continue to ask the same question, the staff will continue to answer that question, and she will continue not to hear their answer. It is too much for anyone to hear.

I used to think that the worst event for a parent was the death of a child. Now I think it is this sort of death-in-life, a condition where the child is gone but not yet dead.

What can we do? I suggest at least trying to consider this patient's mother to be a second patient whose story needs to be heard, who needs to be understood, and who needs whatever therapeutic efforts we can make for her. We could start by making a place and a time for her.

P: Mrs. R, I do need to talk with you. Let me put these charts at the nursing desk, and then let's go sit down for a few minutes. That conference room down the hall is open.

Then:

P: Well, as you see, I don't really have any news for you about John.
R: But is he going to be well? Will he get better?
P: Oh boy! I can imagine, almost, how awful this must be for you.
R: I don't care about me. I just want John to be OK.
P: I know, Mrs. R. Let me see. He's your youngest isn't he?
R: Yes. I have two older daughters.

P: And your husband?

R: John's father?

P: Yes.

R: We've been divorced for 12 years. I never hear from him anymore. John's Dad, that's my second husband, helped raise him. But he's been gone for three years too.

P: So you're it.

R: I'm used to it. I don't care. As long as he gets better.

P: What if he didn't?

R: That can't be. He has to get well.

P: It's terribly important to you.

R: Yes. He has to.

P: And what if . . . ?

R: There's just me and my daughters.

P: You'd miss him terribly.

R: I can't even think of it.

P: I can imagine how hard it is for you when we don't seem to have much hope to hold out.

R: It's terrible. Won't he get better?

P: That's the trouble all right. He probably won't improve much more. This may be all the improvement we'll see.

R: I can't stand it.

I think that this conversation is more on track than the repeated efforts to explain that John isn't improving. This one contains efforts at empathic connections between the new patient (John's mother) and her nurse. But even so, we can expect a return to the prior state of denial and bewilderment. I think this is a good example of a situation where the ordinary caregivers are inadequate to the task and we have to consider expanding the team. A chaplain or pastor, a therapist working with Mrs. R, or sometimes a more distant family member can help her to deal with her loss and her constant pain. In any case, the attention must be toward Mrs. R and her pain, as much as toward John and his condition.

In the end, it is compassion we need. I don't think words are the answer. Perhaps simply sitting with Mrs. R in silence is the best act. Nonverbal behavior may count more than verbal. And humility. We are so powerless in the face of tragedy.

We need compassion for ourselves and our colleagues too. Can you imagine working with patients and families like this day after day? Those who do have my admiration and my gratitude.

Case 52

314 HAS DIARRHEA

It's Sunday at 3 P.M. You have just come home from weekend hospital rounds. The phone rings, and your answering service asks you to call the hospital to talk with Sharon on 3-West about John Jones. You dial the phone number.

S: 3-West, Sharon.
X: Hello, Sharon, this is Dr. X.
S: Oh yeah. Thanks for calling back so quick. 314 has diarrhea.
X: 314?
S: Yeah. That's John Jones. He's Dr. A's patient. You're covering for him?
X: Yes, I am. And I did see Jones when I was there two hours ago. I don't remember the diarrhea though.
S: Yeah. He's had it about a dozen times since last night. He's getting pretty raw, and I wondered if we could give him something for it.
X: Huh! Nobody mentioned it when I was there.
S: Yeah. I might have been on break. Anyway, the aide says he's asking for something for it now.
X: And remind me, why does he have the diarrhea? Is he taking any antibiotics?
S: Just a minute. Let me grab the chart to double-check.

[Long pause; two minutes of hold-music.]

S: Hello, Dr. X?
X: Yes, I'm still here.
S: Sorry, I couldn't find the chart at first. He's on digoxin, potassium, furosemide, zaroxolyn, cefotaxime, timaxin, glyburide, ferrous sulfate, and a bunch of prns.

X: And what was the cefotaxime treating?
S: Just a minute.

[Back on hold; more hold-music.]

R: Hello, this is Ms. Rogers, the nurse manager.
X: What happened to Sharon?
R: She thought you needed me to answer your questions.
X: Oh. Do you know Jones?
R: No, not really. His regular nurse is off today.
X: I guess the question was why he is getting antibiotics?
R: Well they've been stopped. Dr. A stopped the antibiotics Friday.
X: The cefotaxime?
R: Just a minute.
X: No! NO, NO, oh damn!

[More hold-music.]

R: I'm sorry, Doctor. He is still getting the cefotaxime. They stopped the other antibiotics. I think they thought he had pneumonia.
X: And the diarrhea then might be a result of the antibiotics.
R: I suppose so, Doctor. Should we get a C. diff. toxin?
X: Good idea. And would you have someone check his vital signs, including an upright pulse and blood pressure? And see whether there is blood in the stool. And call me back? Don't put me on hold, please. I'll tell you my home number.
R: OK, Doctor.

• Is this an example of team care? Communication between two colleagues? What?
• Are the doctor and the nurses playing in the same field?

Discussion

This doctor and these nurses may be working in different universes. The doctor probably works mostly in the field of diseases. He likes to come to diagnoses before treating problems. These two nurses mostly deal with symptoms. If pressed, they might admit to the value of a better understanding of the patient's disease before treating symptoms, but most of the time they are confronted by bothersome symptoms and used to symptomatic therapy being assigned.

Nurses and sometimes doctors like to say that they work in an entirely different third arena, that of illness and character. Nurses often say that they practice a more holistic sort of health care than do doctors, with more attention to the patient, the person of the patient, and the experience of the illness. And by focusing on symptoms I believe they are partly doing just that. They are at least looking at the matter the same way as their patient. The patient complains of diarrhea; they complain of diarrhea. The idea of a disease entity to be diagnosed and treated is one step away, more of a theoretical abstraction. But it is hard for doctor and nurse to have a very useful conversation until they are talking about the same universe.

Then there's the problem of responsibility. There seems to be nothing like responsibility for avoiding it. I do believe that it is the task of the nurses to keep an eye out for the visiting doctor, to flag the chart if necessary, and to communicate when they are in the same place. If they have missed the doctor when on rounds, the nurse needs to get all the facts before calling. Surely the nurse is going to need to explain current diagnoses, list current medications, and cite current vital signs and observations.

What about the doctor? Well, the first challenge is to remain calm. Stay calm, be patient, and treat the nurse with respect even if it feels as if he or she is not respecting the doctor's process. Then, perhaps, the doctor might mention that he or she does better when called with full information.

Case 53

CONVERSATION FAILURE WINS A PRIZE

Dr. FP: Well, Bruce, I think we're doing all right. Your blood pressure is pretty good, and I think you ought to continue with the same medicines another three months.

B: OK, Fred, that seems right to me.

FP: All right then. I'll see you in three months.

B: Right! How have you been doing?

FP: Pretty good. Actually today was a special day. I just learned that my book on doctor-patient communication won a prize.

B: Really? What book? I didn't know you had written one. What prize?

FP: It's called *Conversation Failure*. The university just gave it their 1993 award for best publication by clinical faculty.

B: That's wonderful. And you say it's about doctor-patient communication?

FP: Yes. It's a series of dialogues that don't go so well.

B: Well, I'm glad you told me. And, you know, hearing this helps me decide about something I was unsure about.

FP: Oh?

B: Yes. I was upset about something that happened last time I was here. And I wasn't sure I wanted to tell you, but knowing what an expert you are on communication, I think maybe I can tell you.

FP: Un-huh. And what was it that happened?

B: Well, I don't know if you remember, but you had a medical student working with you that day, and you sent him in to interview me.

FP: Yes?

B: You hadn't asked my permission. You hadn't introduced him. You just presumed it would be all right with me.

FP: I see.

B: And he was fine, of course, but he did ask fairly intimate questions, and the thing is, I hadn't been asked if it was OK with me.

FP: I see. Hmm.

This man is a clinical psychologist who has been a patient of mine for almost ten years. The events of the last visit were pretty much as he describes them.

- What would you do now?

Discussion

Apologize!

And appreciate the event. There I was, basking in my self-praise, the award from the university, my own pride for a job well done, and my patient's appreciation. If there is a God, she must keep an eye out for opportunities like this. "A quick dose of humility for that fellow!"

"Thanks, I needed that!"

Epilogue

Physicians recognize that some areas will not fall within their competence without special training. As an internist, I am unlikely to do well removing a gallbladder unless I have further surgical training. However I know that I COULD do so, and in the meantime I know people who have such training and am quite content to refer patients who need a cholecystectomy to them. But we have more trouble with processes that we don't seem to be able to refer away, and paramount among them is the matter of conversing with "difficult patients."

The medical literature does identify such patients, but closer study shows that patients who are viewed as difficult by one physician are not so viewed by another. The difficult physician-patient interaction is idiosyncratic and depends on the physician's personality and skills as much as the patient's behavior. We can master techniques to make these difficult interactions manageable.

Are there any adverse side effects from mastering these communication techniques? You bet! I've noticed two. First, my appreciative colleagues say, "Fred really knows how to handle these difficult patients. Let's send him another." Then I get more patients who really take a lot of time, present really difficult relationship problems, and are often more than I can manage on any given day. Second, my friends love to point out to me how badly I have just done at these very procedures that I recommend to others. "Well, big empathy-guru, you really blew that one, didn't you!"

Sic transit gloria mundi.

References

1. Mishler EG. *The Discourse of Medicine* 1984, Ablex, Norwood, NJ.

2. Kleinman A. *The Illness Narratives: Suffering, Healing and the Human Condition* 1988, Basic Books, New York.

3. Berger J, Mohr J. *A Fortunate Man* 1967, Penguin, London.

4. Hopkins GM. "Spring and Fall" in *Poems of Gerard Manley Hopkins* 1948, Oxford University Press, London.

5. Sullivan A. *Pirates of Penzance* in *The Annotated Gilbert and Sullivan* 1982, Harmondsworth, Middlesex, England.

6. Snyder CR, Higgins RL, Stucky RJ. *Excuses, Masquerades in Search of Grace* 1983, Wiley, New York.

7. Dexter C. *The Jewel That Was Ours* 1991, Crown, New York.

8. *A Physician's Guide to Physician-Patient Communication* 1989, The Miles Council for Physician-Patient Communication, West Haven, CT.

9. Platt FW, Carroll JG, Keller V, Gordon GH. Three strategies for improving communication with your patients. *ACP Observer* 1993;13(1):8–10.

10. Platt FW, McMath JC. Clinical hypocompetence: The interview. *Ann Intern Med* 1979;91:898–902.

11. Book HE. Empathy: Misconceptions and misuse in psychotherapy. *Am J Psychiatry* 1988;145:420–424.

12. Brothers L. A biological perspective on empathy. *Am J Psychiatry* 1989;146:10–19.

13. Grattan LM, Eslinger PJ. Empiric study of empathy. *Am J Psychiatry* 1989;146:1521–2.

14. Davis CM. What is empathy, and can empathy be taught? *Phys Ther* 1990;70:707–715.

15. Suchman AL, Mathews DA. What makes the patient-doctor relationship therapeutic? Exploring the connexional dimension of medical care. *Ann Intern Med* 1988;108:125–130.

16. Olsen DP. Empathy as an ethical and philosophical basis for nursing. *Adv Nurs Sci* 1991;14:62–75.

17. Platt FW, Keller VF. Empathic communication, a teachable and learnable skill. *J Gen Intern Med* 1994;9:222–226.

18. Smith RC, Hoppe RB. The patient's story: Integrating the patient- and physician-centered approaches to interviewing. *Ann Intern Med* 1991;115:470–477.

19. Platt FW. Weekend Rounds. In *Conversation Failure* 1992, Life-Sciences Press, Tacoma, WA.

20. Bird J, Cohen-Cole SA. The three function model of the medical interview: An educational device. In M Hale (ed), *Models of Consultation-Liaison Psychiatry* 1990, S. Karger AG, Basel.

21. Cohen-Cole SA. *The Medical Interview: The Three Function Approach,* 1991, Mosby, St. Louis.

22. Lewis CS. *Till We Have Faces: A Myth Retold* 1956, Harcourt, Brace, New York.

23. Williams GC et al. The facts concerning the recent carnival of smoking in Connecticut and elsewhere. *Ann Intern Med* 1991;115:59–63.

24. Herman JL. *Trauma and Recovery* 1992, Basic Books, New York.

25. White MK, Keller V. *Annotated Bibliography: "Difficult"*

Physician-Patient Relationships 1992, Miles Institute for Health Care Communications, West Haven, CT.

26. Lipp MR. *Respectful Treatment: A Practical Handbook of Patient Care* (2nd ed) 1986, Elsevier, New York.

27. Scarlett EP. What Is a Profession? In J Stone and R Reynolds (eds), *On Doctoring* 1991, Simon & Schuster, New York, pp. 119–133.

28. Illich I. *Medical Nemesis: The Expropriation of Health* 1976, Random House, New York.

29. Novack DH et al. Physicians' attitudes toward using deception to resolve difficult ethical problems. *JAMA* 1989;261:2980–2985.

30. Eisenberg DM, et al. Unconventional medicine in the United States: Prevalence, costs, and patterns of use. *N Engl J Med* 1993;328:246–252.

31. Morgan WL Jr, Engel GL. *The Clinical Approach to the Patient* 1969, Saunders, Philadelphia.

32. Weed L. Medical records that guide and teach. *N Engl J Med* 1968;278:593–599, 652–658.

33. Enelow AJ, Swisher SN. *Interviewing and Patient Care* 1986, Oxford University Press, New York.

34. Coulehan JL, Block MR. *The Medical Interview: A Primer for Students of the Art* (2nd ed) 1992, Davis, Philadelphia.

35. Molde S, Baker D. Exploring primary care visits. *Image* 1985;17:72–76.

36. Sheagren JN, Zweifler AJ, Woolliscroft JO. The present medical database needs reorganization: It's time for a change! *Arch Intern Med* 1990;150:2014–2015.

37. Buchsbaum DG, et al. A program of screening and prompting improves short-term physician counseling of dependent and nondependent harmful drinkers. *Arch Intern Med* 1993;153:1573–1577.

38. Ende J, Rockwell S, Glasgow M. The sexual history in gen-

eral internal medicine practice. *Arch Intern Med.* 1984; 144:558–561.

39. HIV prevention practices of primary care physicians— USA—1992. *MMWR* 1993;42:988–992.

40. Smart CR, et al. Cancer Screening and Early Detection. In JF Holland et al. (eds), *Cancer Medicine* 1993, Lea & Febiger, Philadelphia, pp. 408–431.

41. McGoldrick M, Gerson R. Clinical Uses of the Genogram. In *Genograms in Family Assessment* 1985, Norton, New York, pp. 125–160.

42. Beck JC, Freedman ML, Warshaw GA. Geriatric assessment: Focus on function. *Patient Care* 1994;28(4):10–32.

43. Mitchell TL et al. The yield of the screening review of systems. *J Gen Intern Med* 1992;7:393–397.

44. Gordon GH, Dunn P. Advance directives and the patient self-determination act. *Hosp Pract,* April 30, 1992, pp. 39–42.

45. Pfeifer MP et al. The discussion of end-of-life medical care by primary care patients and physicians. *J Gen Intern Med* 1994;9:82–88.

46. Kahana RJ, Bibring GL. Personality Types in Medical Management. In NE Zinberg (ed), *Psychiatry and Medical Practice in a General Hospital* 1964, International University Press, New York, pp. 108–123.

47. Prochaska J, DiClemente C. Stages and processes of self change of smoking: Toward an integrative model of change. *J Consult Clin Psychol* 1983;51(3):390–395.

48. Korsh BM, Gozzi EK, Francis V. Gaps in doctor-patient communication. *Pediatrics* 1968;42:855–871.

49. Beckman HB, Frankel RM. The effect of physician behavior on the collection of data. *Ann Intern Med* 1984;101:692–696.

50. Balint M. *The Doctor, His Patient and the Illness* 1957, International University Press, Madison, CT.

51. Lipp M. *The Bitter Pill: Doctors, Patients, and Failed Expectations* 1980, Harper and Row, New York.

52. Fred HL. The interesting patient. *Hosp Pract*, April 15, 1993, p. 10.

53. Grann V. The interesting patient syndrome. *Arch Intern Med* 1965;116:442–444.

54. Burack RC, Carpenter RR. The predictive value of the presenting complaint. *J Fam Pract* 1983;4:749–754.

Index